Epidemiological Research: Terms and Concepts

O. S. Miettinen

Epidemiological Research: Terms and Concepts

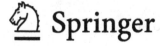 Springer

Prof. Dr. O. S. Miettinen
McGill University
Cornell University
1020 Pine Avenue West
Montrèal, QC H3A 1A2
Canada
olli.miettinen@mcgill.ca

ISBN 978-94-017-8436-8   ISBN 978-94-007-1171-6 (eBook)
DOI 10.1007/978-94-007-1171-6
Springer Dordrecht Heidelberg London New York

Springer is part of Springer Science+Business Media (www.springer.com)

Preface

In his *The Joys of Yiddish* (1970), Leo Rosten delights the reader with this vignette:

> A bright young *chachem* told his grandmother that he was going to be a Doctor of Philosophy. She smiled proudly: 'Wonderful. But what kind of disease is philosophy?'

The reader here might wonder what a chachem is, but not after reading Rosten: it's a great scholar, a clever and wise learned person. On the other hand, though, the reader here, like that grandmother, likely presumes to know what a *doctor* and a *disease* are; but (s)he might do well consulting a suitable source on this too – a contemporary medical dictionary won't do (cf. sect. I – 1. 1 here) – insofar as (s)he is enough of a chachem to really care about the meanings (s)he associates with words.

According to *The American Heritage Dictionary of the English Language*, a dictionary is, in one of the four meanings of the word, "A book listing words or other linguistic items in a particular category of subject with specialized information about them: *a medical dictionary*." The listing generally is alphabetical in its ordering.

This book is, mainly, a dictionary in that meaning, with *terms* of American English – and some of their initials-based abbreviations also – addressed in alphabetical order; but it also is designed – by the proposed selection from among the terms and the proposed ordering of these – to function as a textbook in an introductory course on epidemiological research (see Introduction below). A term is, in logic and also in that word's usage here, a word or a composite of words – such as 'epidemiological research' – that can be the subject or predicate of a proposition [1].

The "specialized information" that this book gives about the terms it covers is their meanings, that is, the *concepts* to which they refer. This information is, in part, merely descriptive of prevailing terms and the concepts to which they refer; but it commonly also is quasi-prescriptive, conveying my opinion of what the term or the concept, or both, ought to be. A concept is the essence of a thing (entity, quality/quantity, relation); it is true of every instance of the thing and unique to it [1].

A concept is specified by its *definition*, which – in an ideal definition at least – posits the concept's "proximate genus" together with its "specific difference" within this genus [1]. For epidemiological research the proximate genus obviously is research; but the specific difference – true of every instance of this research and unique to this particular genre of research – scarcely is a matter of shared understanding among, even, teachers of this research. In this book, many of the definitions are supplemented by explications of their meanings, as I see them – extensive explications, even.

With that "medical dictionary" term as a paradigm, this book can be said to be, in part, an epidemiological-research dictionary. This research is mostly about the causal origin – *etiology, etiogenesis* – of illness, knowledge of which is seen to be critically important for the practice of epidemiology – meaning, of community medicine, community-level (rather than clinical) preventive medicine. For another part, this book is a dictionary of related, meta-epidemiological *clinical research*, for clinical medicine. Both of these address, mostly, *rates* of the occurrence of events and states of ill-health/illness, and therefore clinical researchers, too, now tend to develop their concepts and terms – and principles, even – largely by studying epidemiological research.

Etiologic research has undergone enormous growth in the most recent half-century; and along with this there has been major development also of the very concepts and terms of epidemiological research. Around 1960 it was, still, conceptually unsurprising for an authoritative "committee on design and analysis of studies" [2] to declare that "The ideal epidemiological study would be based on probability samples from a very large population . . . ," even though no-one conducting 'bench research' was dreaming of probability samples of very large populations of particular types of rodents; and it was both conceptually and linguistically unsurprising that a major authority on the theory of epidemiological research classified etiologic studies in the broadest categories of "descriptive" and "analytic" studies [3].

To help epidemiologists keep up with the conceptual and linguistic – English-language – developments concerning epidemiological research, the International Epidemiological Association has been sponsoring *A Dictionary of Epidemiology*, which now is in its fifth edition [4]; but I consider this program to have been less successful than it really could, and should, have been [5, 6]. The examples below should suffice to justify this judgment.

The I.E.A. dictionary defines *etiology* as: "Literally, the science of causes, causality; in common usage, cause." This is all that it says about this central concept in epidemiological research. But if etiology indeed were, "literally," the science of causes (in truth there is no such science, just as morphology, e.g., is not a science), then, for example, tautology would be, literally, the science of unnecessary repetition [7]; and if any given cause of an illness were, in common medical conception, an "etiology" of that illness, then the word 'etiology' would have no justification for inclusion in the lexicons of medicine (in addition to that less abstruse term 'cause'). But the medical concept of etiology actually is, as I let on above, that of causal origin – etiogenesis – of illness [8]; and in respect to any given cause, etiology thus is the role of this cause in the initiation and/or advancement of the genesis of the illness.

That dictionary describes *etiologic study* as being of three common types: "cross-sectional, cohort, and case-control" (*sic*). To the respective definitions of these are associated quite extensive annotations; but none of these is about the fundamental misconceptions that those types of study represent, nor about the linguistic awkwardness of that triad of terms; and there are no words about the necessary, singular essence of etiologic studies that is dictated by logic [7, 9].

Rate – a concept as central as any to etiologic research as well as to the practice of epidemiology (as community medicine) – that dictionary defines as "an expression of the frequency with which an event [*sic*] occurs in a defined population," as though there were no rates for the occurrence of states of illness; that is, it defines rate as though there were no rates of prevalence (of states) in addition to rates of incidence (of events). And indeed, concerning prevalence rate the dictionary declares: "It is a proportion, not a rate." Yet the dictionary presents without any critical annotation "adult literacy rate," "response rate," and "survival rate," for example, each of them a proportion. (Cf., e.g., 'unemployment rate' in general English.)

Such confusion in this context is compounded by faltering logic. For example, while the dictionary says that "All rates are ratios, calculated by dividing a numerator ... by a denominator ... ," the numerator and denominator are said to be "components of a rate" rather than inputs into its calculation; and yet another "component" is said to be "the specified time in which events occur," as though this were not already involved in the inputs into the rate's calculation (insofar as it actually is involved at all; in proportion-type rates it isn't).

Illness – a recurrent concept and term in the foregoing, already, as it too is very central – the I.E.A. dictionary addresses under "disease" only. What it there says does not reflect familiarity with these two concepts and terms in medicine, including awareness of the confusion about them that now prevails even in eminent, "authoritative" dictionaries of medicine [10, 11].

Illness, I propose, should be understood to be any ill-health, and the term thus to be the English-language counterpart of *Krankheit* in German and *maladie* in French. Disease (L. *morbus*) in the medical usage of the term is but one of the principal subtypes of illness, the others being defect (L. *vitium*) and injury (Gr. *trauma*) – as has been explained elsewhere [10, 11], without any objection from the I.E.A. or any other source.

Epidemiological research is, by the very nature of its objects, *statistical* research; and as such, it commonly is testing of etiologic hypotheses. The central statistic now derived from the data of such studies is the null P-value. The I.E.A. dictionary defines *P-value*, in the meaning of the null P-value, as: "The probability that a test statistic would be as extreme as observed or more extreme if the null hypothesis were true." This conception of the essence of the null P-value – with probability taken to be its proximate genus – is quite unfortunate, even though very common. For, it underpins the common, serious misconception that the null P-value is the probability that the 'null hypothesis' is true.

A preferable conception of the null P-value, ignored in the I.E.A. dictionary, is this [12]: a statistic so derived that on the 'null hypothesis' its distribution is uniform in the 0-to-1 range – so that $\Pr(P < \alpha) = \alpha$ – and that, in addition, on the hypothesis proper (when the 'null hypothesis' is not true) its distribution, still within the 0-to-1 range, is shifted to the left – so that $\Pr(P < \alpha) > \alpha$. At issue is the very same statistic as is addressed by the I.E.A. dictionary definition, but now defined in terms of its intended distribution, analogously with the way a 'confidence interval' generally is conceptualized and defined. With this definition of the null P-value there is no propensity to think of it as the probability that the 'null hypothesis' is true.

When a dictionary of epidemiology is I.E.A.-sponsored, it shouldn't commonly be questionable or even definitely wrong in its contents, the central ones in particular; for this does not promote sound development of the theory – concepts, principles, and terminology – of epidemiological research [5, 6]. In fact, any dictionary of epidemiology that claims to be authoritative – as the I.E.A. dictionary has done, its current Editor describing it as representing "a high level of scientific and intellectual rigor" (Preface) – may even retard progress. It may stifle critical reflection on the terms and concepts it presents.

For optimal development of the terms and concepts specific to epidemiological *research*, needed is, first, an alternative dictionary, periodically updated, in which the content is presented in the spirit of *propositions*, for the community of epidemiological researchers not simply to believe (or contradict) but to "weigh and consider" – the readers thus heeding an important precept of Francis Bacon on how to read [13]. I compiled this dictionary in response to that need, still otherwise unfulfilled.

The next need is for pursuit and attainment of practical *consensus* about the thus-presented terms and concepts in the community of the researchers. For, as Isaiah Berlin put it [14],

> where the concepts are firm, clear and generally accepted, and the methods of reasoning and arriving at conclusions are agreed between men (at least the majority of those who have anything to do with these matters), there and only there is it possible to construct a science, formal or empirical.

This insight applies to epidemiological research as well, even though this research does not constitute a science unto itself but is, instead, imbedded in various medical sciences – neuroscience/neurology and cardiology, for example.

With possible terms and concepts of epidemiological research put forward as propositions for the researchers to weigh and consider, they are intended to constitute a starting point for the development of consensus about the terms and concepts – through *public discourse* about them. This discourse naturally is a matter of public presentations of criticisms about the propositions, for a start; and these criticisms need to be responded to in a manner more constructive than that of the current Editor of the I.E.A. dictionary [15].

For that public discourse to really take place, extensively and in a timely fashion, there should be formed and maintained a *forum* dedicated to this, somewhere in cyberspace. At issue would be, as in this dictionary, *general terms and concepts*, exclusive of those specific to particular areas of subject-matter of the research. (The

I.E.A. dictionary addresses some of the latter, thus only nibbling at the enormous number of terms and concepts of epidemiological research across the various disciplines of medicine.)

Epidemiological research is concretely purposive – rather than merely interest-driven – when its aim is to advance the *knowledge-base* – scientific – of the practice of epidemiology – of community medicine, that is. Such research is quintessentially 'applied' [16]. It addresses rates, etiologically and otherwise; for, rates of the occurrence of illness are the objects of the practice of epidemiology: the practitioner's concerns are to know about them in the cared-for population and, then, to control them (by the means of community-level preventive medicine).

The knowledge-base of (the practice of) *clinical* medicine is not about rates but about probabilities [16]; but research on probabilities is about (probability-implying) rates. Therefore, quintessentially 'applied' clinical research is *meta-epidemiological* in nature, and it thus has become a concern of teachers of epidemiological research [16, 17]. It is a concern in the I.E.A. dictionary, and so it also is here.

"In a man's life dreams always precede deeds. Perhaps this is because, as Goethe said, 'Our desires are presentiments of the faculties latent within us and signs of what we may be capable of doing . . . we crave for what we already secretly possess. Passionate anticipation thus changes that which is materially possible into dreamed reality' " [18].

In my life ever since medical-school graduation half-a-century ago, I've had the dream of reaching true understanding of the theory of the research that would best serve to advance the knowledge-base of medicine, of genuinely scientific medicine [16, 19]. Having devoted my entire career to this pursuit, I've been craving, all along, for access to genuinely scholarly dictionaries of medicine, both clinical and community medicine, and of directly practice-serving medical research, both clinical and community-medical research. But these dreams have not really come true, to what I'd consider a reasonable approximation.

In an effort to make the dreamed reality come closer in respect to epidemiological research and meta-epidemiological clinical research also, I now launch this dictionary as the initial step. But the reality actually will have come about only when all of the orientational issues addressed in the foregoing, and numerous others, have been brought to secure closure – tentatively at least – by public discourse among epidemiological and clinical researchers and – not to be forgotten – those whose careers are dedicated, in part at least, to the advancement and teaching of the theory of epidemiological and/or related clinical research.

In the meantime, students of epidemiological research need to critically weigh and consider the terms and concepts – or concepts and terms – of epidemiological research as these are being taught, even if the teaching be done by the most senior of epidemiologic academics (myself included [17]).

Introduction

The I.E.A. dictionary [4] addresses almost 2,000 terms and, of course, the meanings of these. Those beginning with A run from *Abatement* to *Axis*, the B-terms from *Background level, rate* to *Burden of disease*, the C-terms from *Calibration* to *Cyst count*, ...

From presentations like this, so William James taught, "We carve out order by leaving the disorderly parts out." I leave out, for example, "*Age* The WHO recommends that age should be defined by completed units of time, counting the day of birth as zero"; "*Gender* 1. In grammar, ... 2. The totality of culturally constructed ... about males and females and sometimes their sexual orientation"; "*GDP* Gross domestic product"; "*Goal* A desired state to be achieved within a specified time"; "*Interval* The set containing all numbers between two given numbers"; "*Justice* 1. A morally defensible distribution of benefits and rewards in society. ... 2. In law, the successful administration of the rule of law"; and "*Sex ratio* The ratio of one sex to the other."

As another means to enhance order, I organize the terms and concepts into three main parts of this book, only one of these focusing on epidemiological research proper. This expressly epidemiologic part is preceded by one with separate sections for *medicine, science* in general, and *statistics* as plain statistics; and this epidemiologic part is followed by a related one, specific to *meta-epidemiological clinical* research.

Moreover, in the two parts focusing on the research that is expressly at issue here, I invoke a further measure to counteract entropy – chaos – of concepts. I arrange to have three separate sections within each of them: one of them covers select introductory terms and concepts, another one is more-or-less specific to *objects* of study, and the third one is more-or-less specific to *methods* of the research.

The coverage here is not confined to what remains from the entries in the I.E.A. dictionary. But where the topic is addressed in that other dictionary as well, this is indicated by an asterisk attached to the term, for the reader to be able to know that what is presented here is a second opinion to that expressed in the I.E.A. dictionary, a second opinion that may not accord with that first opinion.

When a dictionary of epidemiological (and meta-epidemiological clinical) research is organized in this way, its use as a handbook (à la I.E.A. dictionary) can be challenging due to uncertainty about where – in which one(s) of the sections – the term can be found. To obviate this, a single Index at the end of this book lists all of the terms in the alphabetical order, and for each of them it gives the section reference(s) for the definition (and whatever Notes may be associated with it).

Relevant, well-formed concepts and the appropriate terms to express them are the essence of the contents in an ***introductory course*** on epidemiological (and meta-epidemiological clinical) research [17]; and this leads to a particular concern in the ordering of the topics, one that is central to philosophy: Chief among Aristotle's enormous accomplishments has been seen to be the establishment of the basis for correct thinking in terms of the rules of logic (*analytika)* that also enable discourse (*logos*) to become most productive – given also the development of suitable language for use as an enabling instrument of thought with a logically ordered structure and for the expression of this. And Kant's central thesis – very productive – was that the human mind confers a structure for knowledge through the concepts ("categories") that it brings to the acquisition of experience and to learning from it. In line with these extraordinarily fruitful ideas, Robert Roberts and W. Jay Wood in their *Intellectual Virtues* (2007) make the point that, "The real goal of philosophy, perhaps unachievable but still ideal, is reduction, the derivation of all the concepts in a given field from a single, key concept."

In this book, obviously, the introductory key concepts are those of medicine, science, and statistics; and then comes the core concept, the essence of epidemiological research, which is extended to that of meta-epidemiological clinical research. In an introductory course nominally addressing epidemiological research, the teacher would do well placing this research in its context, defining all five of those key concepts; and (s)he needs to try to follow a *logical sequence* in the introduction of the concepts of epidemiological, and of meta-epidemiological clinical, research, endeavoring to 'deduce' the subordinate concepts, sequentially, from the core concept.

I offer a suggestion for the sequence of the concepts' entry into an introductory course on epidemiological research. This I do in what follows the Index: Hierarchy of Concepts.

Acknowledgements

Miguel Porta had a major role in inspiring me to take on the task of developing this first edition of a new dictionary of epidemiological research, as an alternative to the dictionary now being published, in successive editions, by the International Epidemiological Association, with Porta the current Editor [4]. I really am very grateful to him, however unwitting may have been his inspirational role [15].

Given the total agenesis of my keyboard-related skills, *Rebecca Fuhrer*, my Departmental Chairperson, arranged for the requisite help. This was provided by *Kierla Ireland* in the main, with great skill and dedication, and with good cheer to boot. These two persons' role in this book's development was critical, and I much appreciate it.

Some local colleagues read a near-final draft of this book, and I am grateful for their suggestions – those of *Igor Karp* and *James Hanley* in particular.

In due deference to a giant of "the proper study of mankind" (I. Berlin; [14]), I underscored above (in the Preface) the importance of pursuing convergence of the concepts of epidemiological research to generally agreed-upon ones, and of the use of apposite terms also. And to this end, so I said, there should be public discourse among epidemiological researchers and the theoreticians of their work. For an undelayed opener of that discourse, I asked four highly esteemed colleagues to produce commentaries on a near-final draft of this book. These colleagues were: *James Hanley* (development and teaching, especially, of the statistics of epidemiological and clinical research), *Albert Hofman* (practice and teaching of epidemiological and clinical research, and editing a journal of epidemiology), *Andrew Miles* (philosophy of public health and editing a journal on clinical medicine in public health), and *Dimitrios Trichopoulos* (practice and teaching of epidemiological research and book-editing on teaching of epidemiology). They were, of course, free to engage co-authors of their own choosings. Their commentaries presumably will appear in the fullness of time, locus yet to be determined.

Insofar as some of these colleagues will respond to this call for public discourse, they will act the way genuine scholars do act, on this level already. But more to the point, they presumably will do so upon having read the draft of this book in the spirit which Francis Bacon counseled all of us to adopt: "Read not to contradict, nor to believe, but to weigh and consider" [13]. They thus will make a notable contribution to the mission here, and for this I thank them in advance already – on behalf of epidemiological researchers at large.

Contents

PART I
MEDICINE, SCIENCE,
AND STATISTICS

I – 1. TERMS AND CONCEPTS OF MEDICINE

I – 1. 1. Introduction

The concept of *medicine* is defined with "art" as its proximate genus in one of the two most eminent – "authoritative" – English-language dictionaries of medicine, but with "art and science" in this role in the other; and as the specific differences within these genera the two dictionaries give the respective concerns, "preventing or curing disease" and "the diagnosis and treatment of disease and the maintenance of health" [20]. The I.E.A. dictionary [4] leaves medicine undefined.

Critically examined, medicine can be seen to indeed be *art*, in the Aristotelian meaning of 'art' (that of a 'productive art' of making things, as distinct from science, producing knowledge – *epistēmē*); but it never is science [21]. It no longer is *the* art of anything, as modern medicine already is differentiated into scores of component arts – disciplines, 'specialties' – of medicine [22]; and continuing progress will only accentuate this differentiation. (When no one can be a generalist, no one is a specialist either. Cf. professional engineers, musicians, athletes, . . .)

The arts/disciplines of medicine fall in two broad categories. Most of them are disciplines of *clinical* medicine, the others being ones of *community* medicine. The latter segment of medicine is alternatively termed *epidemiology* (or social medicine, or preventive medicine). The definitional distinction between the clinical and epidemiological disciplines has to do with the generic nature of the physicians' client(s). A clinician's clients are individuals, cared for one at a time, while an epidemiologist has a particular population as his/her single client.

Medicine is *healthcare* provided by a physician to his/her client(s). The essence of this care is not "preventing or curing disease," nor "treatment of disease and the maintenance of health"; for, far from always being a feature of physician-provided healthcare, these actions are (highly) exceptional even in the practice of modern medicine, most notably as writing a prescription for a therapeutic medication is but an authorization and instruction for the client (in this case a patient) to execute the treatment.

In providing healthcare, a physician's first concern always necessarily is to get to *know* about the client's health (the client may not be a patient even in clinical medicine), to know about this more specifically and/or more deeply than is possible for the laity. Having attained such esoteric knowing – *gnosis* (dia-, etio-, and/or prognosis) – about the client's health, a physician's – doctor's – responsibility and role is to *teach*, whenever possible, the client (or the client's representatives) accordingly (L. *doctor*, 'teacher'). These two functions of doctors, and these alone, constitute the definitional essence of medicine (i.e., they are always involved in, and unique to, medicine; cf. Preface).

Medical research, while not definitional to medicine (as medicine is not a science), is not even an occasional element in medicine. It thus is not research *in* medicine: epidemiological research is not community medicine, nor is clinical research clinical medicine; these are research *for* community and clinical medicine, respectively.

Even though there now are some tendencies to extend the concepts of both 'epidemiological' and 'clinical' research beyond that of expressly medical research, no-one denies that both types of research are medical in part at least. In this book, both epidemiological and meta-epidemiological clinical research are viewed only from the vantage of medical research; and whereas the researcher may not have a medical background, an introduction into the here-essential terms and concepts of medicine per se also is called for. An added reason for addressing the terms and concepts of medicine per se is the still quite sketchy development of these terms and concepts even within medicine, as is manifest in today's dictionaries of medicine (cf. concept of medicine itself above). Some of these terms and concepts are addressed in the I. E. A. dictionary as well.

I – 1. 2. Mini-dictionary

Where an asterisk (*) is here attached to a term, it indicates the term's inclusion in the I.E.A. dictionary of epidemiology [4].

Abnormal (antonym: normal) – See 'Normal.'

Acquired (antonym: congenital) – Concerning an illness (a case of it or the illness at large), the quality of being postnatal in origin (rather than congenital).

Acute* (antonym: chronic) – Concerning a sickness or an illness, or an epidemic, the quality of being (abrupt, rather than insidious, in onset and) of short duration.

Adjusted rate* – See 'Rate' (Note 6).

Aetiology* – See 'Etiogenesis.'

Agent* – Concerning a sickness or an illness, an extrinsic factor involved in its very definition (as in the case of, e.g., protein sickness, radiation sickness, tuberculosis, asbestosis, and silicosis); also: an extrinsic etiogenetic factor – cause – of a sickness or illness (e.g., ionizing radiation or heat as the agent in the etiogenesis of a burn).

Note: *M. tuberculosis* is not a/the cause of tuberculosis; nor is asbestos a/the cause of asbestosis, silica a/the cause of silicosis, etc. For in these examples the agent is definitional to the illness [23].

Anamnesis – In the pursuit of diagnosis in clinical medicine, the history and status ascertained by interview of the client/patient. (Gr. *anamnesis*, 'recalling.') (Cf. 'History.')

Anomaly – In a person's soma, a marked abnormality (of structure and/or function).
    Note: An abnormal test result, even if markedly abnormal, is not generally termed an anomaly.

Assessment (synonym: estimation) – Concerning something quantitative, development of a view about its level/magnitude. (Examples: assessment/estimation of fitness to undergo thoracotomy and lobectomy of a lung; and assessment/estimation of left-ventricular ejection-fraction in the light of, i.a., the result of an ultrasonic measurement of it.) (Cf. 'Evaluation' and 'Measurement.')
    Note: By the nature of assessment/estimation, *judgment* is generally involved in the development of the result. (Cf. 'assessment' of the market value of a home.)

At risk – Concerning a person's future in respect to coming down with a particular sickness or illness, the quality of being seen to be – by whatever assessment – at non-zero risk for it. (Cf. 'Candidate.')
    Note: Only a person not having a particular sickness or illness can be viewed as being at risk for it.

*Attributable** – Concerning a phenomenon of health (possibly a component of the rate of morbidity from a particular illness) in relation to a particular, potentially etiogenetic factor, the quality of the former of actually having been caused by the latter.

Candidate – A person for whom a particular action (medical) is a realistic option; also: a person who could come down with a particular illness by virtue of being at risk for it. (Examples: Any woman is a candidate for developing uterine cancer so long as she is not in status post hysterectomy; and if she has been diagnosed with a case of uterine cancer, she commonly is a candidate for hysterectomy as the treatment for it.)

Care – See 'Healthcare.'

*Case** – Concerning a sickness or an illness (or whatever else), an instance of it.
    Note: A person with a case of an illness is not a case of that illness; and a number of cases of an illness is not a group but a *series* of these (in a group of people).

*Case-fatality rate** (synonyms: fatality rate, death rate) – Concerning cases of an illness in general, or recognized cases of it (ones with rule-in diagnosis about the

illness), the proportion in which the illness is fatal; that is, such that the outcome of
the course of the illness is fatality from it. (Cf. 'Survival rate.')

Note: For the concept to be truly meaningful, it commonly is to be *specific* to
particulars of the case (broadly at least) and to the choice of treatment; and it also
is to be *conditional* on absence of intercurrent death from some other, 'competing'
cause.

*Case finding** – Given a recognized point source of exposure to an agent definitional
or causal to a sickness or an illness (see 'Agent'), the pursuit of case identification
among persons known or suspected to have had that particular exposure.

*Catchment area** – Concerning a particular type of care from the vantage of a
particular facility for the care, or set of such facilities, the area (geographic or
jurisdictional) from which (at least most of) the persons receiving that care come.

Note: The concept is meaningful only if meant is the smallest population of this
type (rather than, e.g., the world population at large).

Catchment population – Concerning a particular type of care from the vantage of
a particular facility for the care, or set of such facilities, the population (of people)
from which (at least most of) the persons receiving that care come.

Note: See Note under 'Catchment area.'

*Cause** – Concerning a particular aspect of health in the abstract, a thing the presence of which can produce an effect on – a change in – it, change that would not
be produced by the defined alternative to this thing. By the same token, concerning
health in a particular instance (of a person or a population), a thing that did, or will,
produce an effect – a change – in it, change that would not have happened, or would
not happen, in the presence of its alternative (specified).

Note 1: While, in a sense, papilloma virus is a cause of cervical cancer and
H. pylori is a cause of peptic ulcer, *M. tuberculosis* is not a/the cause of tuberculosis nor is asbestos a/the cause of asbestosis, etc.; nor is a bullet ever causal to a
bullet wound, a poison causal to poisoning, etc.: When something becomes definitional to an illness or a sickness, it can no longer (logically) be a/the cause of it (cf.
Note under 'Agent'); now the proximal causes are presence of that something (constitutional, behavioral, or environmental) and susceptibility to contract the illness or
sickness from this presence.

Contributing cause – Concerning a particular case (of sickness, illness, or death),
a cause other than the one principally at issue, one that also was present and was
critical for the causation principally at issue.

Note 2: The presence of a contributing cause does not make the one principally
at issue less of a cause: both had a critical role (*ceteris paribus*).

Underlying cause – Concerning a particular case (of sickness, illness, or death),
a cause of the cause principally at issue, one that also was present and was causal to
the cause principally at issue. Example: Given cerebrovascular hemorrhage as the
proximal cause of a stroke, an underlying cause may be 'hypertension' (this term is
a misnomer for high blood-pressure).

Ceteris paribus – All else (that is relevant) being equal.

*Chronic** (antonym: acute) – Concerning a sickness or an illness, or an epidemic, the quality of being of long duration. (Cf. 'Subacute.')

Client – In relation to a particular physician, a/the recipient of care from him/her.
   Note 1: A clinical physician's client (in a given encounter) may not be a patient; and the client of a community physician never is. (See 'Patient.')
   Note 2: Different from lawyers, for example, doctors eschew the term 'client,' preferring 'patient' (i.e., being unique in this way).

Clinical – Concerning healthcare, the quality of having to do with individuals, one at a time (as distinct from epidemiological care, for a population); also: concerning a case of an illness, the quality of it being overt, manifest in sickness; and concerning gnosis in clinical medicine, the quality of it being based, in its ad-hoc inputs, solely on non-laboratory items. (Gr. *klinikos*, 'bed.')

Clinical diagnosis – See 'Clinical' and 'Diagnosis.'

*Clinical epidemiology** – A generally self-contradictory term for a still-inchoate but nevertheless manifestly malformed concept [16]. (See 'Medicine' and Note 2 under 'Public health'.)
   Note 1: The I.E.A. dictionary [4] defines clinical epidemiology as: "The application of epidemiological knowledge, reasoning, and methods to study clinical issues and improve clinical care." (See 'Evidence-Based Medicine' and 'Professionalism.')
   Note 2: Were there justifiably to be the concept of clinical epidemiology, there presumably would also be that of epidemiological clinical medicine (à la medical science vis-à-vis scientific medicine [19]) – but there hasn't been, nor should there be.

Clinical etiognosis – See 'Clinical' and 'Etiognosis.'

Clinical medicine – See 'Medicine.'

Clinical prognosis – See 'Clinical' and 'Prognosis.'

Clinician – A physician who works directly – as at the bedside – with individual clients. (Example: an anesthesiologist.) (Gr. *klinikos*, 'bed.')
   Note 1: Among physicians who deal with individual clients (in clinical medicine), many do not work directly with them – pathologists and most radiologists, for example. These physicians are not clinicians.
   Note 2: In a given encounter (direct) with a client, a clinician may not act as the client's doctor; an anesthesiologist, for example, generally doesn't. (See 'Doctor'; L. *doctor*, 'teacher.')

*Community diagnosis** – See 'Diagnosis.'

Community etiognosis – See 'Etiognosis.'

*Community health** – The aggregate of disciplines, medical and paramedical, concerned with control of morbidity (in a community/population); also: the work of this aggregate of disciplines in caring for their client community/population. (Cf. 'Public health.')

Note: 'Health' is here substituted for 'medicine' so as to be inclusive of paramedical disciplines and their work.

*Community medicine** – See 'Medicine.'

Community prognosis – See 'Prognosis.'

*Comorbidity** – The presence, in an individual, of an illness, or illnesses, other than the one at issue.

Note: This term, recently introduced into clinical medicine via 'clinical epidemiology,' is a misnomer for its referent. The corresponding appropriate terms would be 'co-illness' and 'co-illnesses' (cf., e.g., 'co-author'). An individual with a case of some illness doesn't thereby have a case of 'morbidity,' possibly with 'comorbidity' to boot, nor will (s)he ever undergo 'mortality' (even though [s]he is mortal). Morbidity and mortality are concepts of community medicine, not of clinical medicine; and in any client population of community medicine there generally is a large variety of morbidities from particular illnesses, with no reason to think of the aggregate of the others as constituting 'comorbidity' for a given one of the illness-specific morbidities.

*Competing cause** – Concerning potential death from a particular cause, another cause of death capable of averting such a death by causing death before it.

*Compliance** – A patient's (or other client's) adherence to a doctor-prescribed regimen of intervention.

Note: This term and concept, not yet quite passé, relate to doctors' *orders*; but in modern terms, doctors are not supposed to give orders, as the decision-maker is supposed to be understood to be the patient (or other client, suitably informed by the doctor).

Complication – Given a disease or an injury, another illness caused by it; also: given an intervention, an illness caused by it. (Examples: peritonitis as a complication of peptic ulcer; an infection as a complication of an injury; hemorrhagic stroke as a complication of anticoagulation; and cardiac arrest as a complication of anesthesia.) (Cf. 'Sequela.')

Congenital (antonym: acquired) – Concerning an illness, a case of it or of the illness at large, the quality of being prenatal in origin (rather than acquired).

Contra-indication – Concerning a medical action (gnostic or interventive), an indication pointing to adverse consequence(s) of this and thereby being more-or-less prohibitive of the action. (Cf. 'Indication.')

Contributing cause – See 'Cause' (Note 1).

Correct diagnosis/etiognosis/prognosis – See 'Diagnosis'/'Etiognosis'/'Prognosis.'

Course – Concerning a case of a sickness or illness, the way it evolves over time (so long as the evolvement is not interrupted by intercurrent death from some other cause).

Crude rate* – See 'Rate' (Note 5).

Cumulative incidence* – See 'Rate' (Note 4).

Curative – Concerning an intervention, the quality of having the ability to produce cure, or actually having produced cure.
    Note: Clinical medicine is sometimes referred to as curative medicine, thus distinguishing it from preventive medicine, equated with community medicine. But it deserves note that the attainment of cure still is very uncommon in clinical medicine, and that much of preventive medicine actually is clinical.

Cure – A person's complete recovery from (a case of) an illness; also: an action that served, or serves, to bring about complete recovery from an illness. (See 'Outcome.')

Death rate* (synonyms: fatality rate, case-fatality rate) – See 'Case-fatality rate.'
    Note: While the term – one of clinical medicine – is also used as a synonym for mortality rate in community medicine, it would better be Ockham's-razored out of this usage.

Defect – See 'Illness.'

Determinant* – Concerning the probability of a health phenomenon (event or state, in an individual) or the level of a morbidity (in a population), something on which this depends (causally or acausally). (Examples: age and gender per se, as distinct from a particular age or a particular gender, as determinants of short-term risk for myocardial infarction.)

Diagnosed – Concerning a case of illness, the quality of having been associated with a rule-in diagnosis.

Diagnosing (synonym: diagnosticating) – Pursuing diagnosis; also: setting (specifying) diagnosis (in clinical medicine the probability in this) for a particular illness.

*Diagnosis** – A doctor's esoteric knowing (attainable only by doctors) about a/the client's health status, present or past, specifically in respect to a particular illness. (Cf. 'Etiognosis' and 'Prognosis' and see 'Overdiagnosis'):

Clinical diagnosis – A clinical doctor's knowing (esoteric) about the presence/absence, present or past, of a particular illness in a client; also: a clinician's diagnosis based on 'clinical' indicators alone (exclusive of laboratory test results, from imaging, say).

Note 1: Clinical diagnosis, in either one of these meanings, is knowing (esoteric) about the *correct probability* that the illness is/was present (or absent), given the diagnostic profile of the case. *Correct diagnosis* is characterized by this probability, which represents the proportion of instances of the diagnostic profile in general (in the abstract) such that the illness at issue is present [16]. That proportion is the profile-specific general rate of *prevalence* of the illness at issue, implied by a suitable diagnostic prevalence/probability function [16].

Note 2: *Pattern recognition* – recognition of the pattern of manifestations as constituting a *syndrome* and thus being definitional to a particular illness (as generally is the case with mental 'illnesses'/'disorders'/ syndromes) – is not diagnosis (clinical).

Note 3: A patient does not have a diagnosis; only the doctor may have.

Note 4: It remains commonplace to conflate the concepts of clinical rule-in diagnosis about an illness and a case of the illness per se, even though their respective domains are very different (the doctor's mind vs. the patient's body).

*Community diagnosis** – A community doctor's – epidemiologist's – knowing (esoteric) about the level of morbidity, present or past, from a particular illness in the cared-for (client) population.

Diagnostic – Concerning a test, the quality of pertaining to the pursuit of diagnosis; also: a diagnostic test; and further: concerning a symptom or sign, or a cluster of these (i.e., a diagnostic profile), the quality of being pathognomonic about a particular illness.

Diagnosticating (synonym: diagnosing) – See 'Diagnosing.'

Note: 'Diagnosticating' as a synonym for 'diagnosing' is a here-proposed neologism, patterned after 'prognosticating.'

Diagnostic profile – In clinical medicine, the set of (ad-hoc) facts on the basis of which a corresponding diagnosis is to be set (by bringing general medical knowledge to bear). (Cf. 'Diagnosis,' Note 1.)

*Direct standardization** – See 'Rate' (Note 8).

*Disease** – See 'Illness.'

*Disorder** – An occasional synonym for illness (mainly among psychiatrists and 'clinical epidemiologists').

Note: As 'order' is not used, nor deserving of use, as a synonym of 'health' in the meaning of freedom from ill-health/illness, 'disorder' is not an apt synonym for 'illness.'

Doctor – A physician who practices medicine (clinical or community medicine).

Note: Many clinicians do not practice what clinical medicine by definition (of its essence) is, nor do many practicing epidemiologists practice what epidemiology – community medicine – by definition is (see 'Medicine'); that is, they aren't doctors in the genuine meaning of this word. (L. *doctor*, 'teacher.')

*Dose-response** – Concerning the effect of a causal factor, the way in which the magnitude of an/the effect depends on the level of the factor; also: an effect's magnitude being dependent (in whatever way) on the level of the causal factor (but especially so that the effect increases with increasing level of the factor).

Early detection / diagnosis* – Attainment of rule-in diagnosis (about a case of an illness) when the illness still is in the latent – preclinical – stage of its development. (Cf. 'Case finding' and 'Screening.')

*EBM** – Evidence-Based Medicine.

*Effect** – A change produced by a cause, change that would not have occurred, or would not occur, in the presence of its alternative (*ceteris paribus*). (See 'Cause.')

*Effectiveness** (synonym: efficacy) – See 'Efficacy.'

*Efficacy** (synonym: effectiveness) – Concerning an intervention in healthcare, the extent to which it actually has its intended effect, how commonly and/or how strongly. (Cf. 'Safety,' and 'Effectiveness' and 'Efficacy' in sect. III – 2.)

*Endemic** – Concerning a particular population's morbidity from a particular illness at a particular time, the quality of its level being what is usual for that population, more-or-less.

*Epidemic** – Concerning a particular population's morbidity from a particular illness at a particular time, the quality of its level being, temporarily, substantially higher than what is usual for that population; also: a temporary substantial increase in the rate of morbidity from a particular illness in a particular population.

Note: A modern 'epidemiologist' is, typically, more of an *endemiologist* than an actual epidemiologist, literally speaking. Infectious-disease epidemiologists still are the ones most true to the etymologic meaning of 'epidemiologist.' Epidemics are, however, of concern also in the practice of cancer epidemiology, for example.

*Epidemiologist** – A physician who practices community medicine.

*Epidemiology** – Community medicine. See 'Medicine.'

*Estimation** (synonym: assessment) – See 'Assessment.'

Etiogenesis (synonym: etiology) – Concerning a case of an illness, or a rate of occurrence of an illness, its causal origin (in the case of a disease or defect, specifically, the causation of the inception and/or progression of its pathogenesis); also: concerning a sickness or an illness in general (in the abstract), its causal origin in general. (Cf. 'Iatrogenesis' and 'Pathogenesis.')

Note: 'Etiogenesis' – a recent neologism [8] – rhymes with its closely-related semi-cognate 'pathogenesis' – while 'etiology' is prone to be misunderstood (cf. Preface).

Etiogenetic fraction (synonym: etiologic fraction) – Concerning morbidity from a particular illness, in a particular population at a particular time (or possibly in general), in relation to a particular factor/cause, the proportion of the (rate of) morbidity that is attributable (causally) to that factor/cause (its presence in lieu of its alternative).

Note: The EF is the proportion of cases of the illness with the antecedent potential cause multiplied by (RR-1)/RR, where RR is the causal rate-ratio [24].

Etiognosing (synonym: etiognosticating) – Pursuing etiognosis; also: setting (specifying) etiognosis. (Cf. 'Diagnosing.')

Note 1: 'Etiognosing' is a here-proposed neologism, patterned after 'diagnosing.'

Note 2: As of now, knowing about the etiogenesis of a case of an illness is still generally subsumed under diagnosis – despite the profound difference between the *what* and the *why*, here as in general, with etiogenesis still a novel concept [25].

Etiognosis – A doctor's esoteric knowing about the etiogenesis of a patient's case of a particular illness or the cared-for population's level of morbidity for a particular illness, specifically in respect to a particular potential cause:

Clinical etiognosis – A clinical doctor's knowing (esoteric) about the etiogenesis of a patient's illness (with rule-in dgn.) in respect to a particular, potentially etiogenetic antecedent that was there, specifically about whether this antecedent actually caused this case of the illness; also: such etiognosis based on 'clinical' indicators alone (exclusive of laboratory ones). (Even a layperson knows that something that wasn't there wasn't causal.)

Note 1: Clinical etiognosis in either one of these meanings is knowing about the *correct probability* that the antecedent was causal – etiogenetic – to the case at issue. *Correct etiognosis* is characterized by this probability, which represents the proportion of instances of the etiognostic profile (cum the illness and the antecedent) in general such that the antecedent is causal to the illness. (That proportion is implied by a suitable etiognostic probability function [16].)

Community etiognosis – A community doctor's – epidemiologist's – knowing (esoteric) about the etiogenesis of the cared-for population's morbidity, specifically about the extent to which its morbidity from a particular illness is due to a particular factor. It is knowing about the *etiogenetic fraction/proportion* for this cause in the morbidity at issue in the cared-for population at the time. (That proportion is determined by how common is antecedent presence of the factor in persons with the illness, together with the etiognostic probability in these cases [24].)

Note 2: 'Etiognosis' is a recent neologism [25], patterned after 'diagnosis' and 'prognosis.'

Etiognosticating (synonym: etiognosing) – See 'Etiognosing.'
Note: 'Etiognosticating' is a here-proposed neologism, patterned after 'prognosticating.' See Note 2 under 'Etiognosing.'

*Etiologic fraction** (synonyms: etiologic/etiogenetic proportion) – See 'Etiogenetic fraction.'

*Etiologic proportion** (synonyms: etiologic/etiogenetic fraction) – See 'Etiogenetic fraction.'

*Etiology** (synonym: etiogenesis) – See 'Etiogenesis.'

*Evaluation** – Concerning the quality of something, passing judgment on it.
Note 1: Evaluation usually is *subjective*, the judgment expressed on an ordinal scale of (subjective) preference, such as: excellent/good/fair/poor.
Note 2: Given a generally agreed-upon scale of quality (of an aspect of healthcare, say), evaluation is assessment (quasi-objective) on this scale.
Note 3: In clinical jargon, *any assessment* is commonly (though unjustifiably) termed evaluation.

*Evidence-Based Medicine** – A purported "new paradigm" for the practice of clinical medicine, adduced in the early 1990s, in which deference to experts is replaced by practitioners' own, critical reading of original literature and its reviews [26]. "Clinical epidemiology" is said to be the "basic science" of EBM, which now is defined by its leaders as "the integration of best research evidence with clinical expertise and patient values" [27]. A whole body of precepts [27] – commonly quite objectionable [16] – constitutes the ideology of this movement. (Cf. 'Knowledge-based medicine.')

Expert – In medicine, a physician with an outstandingly high level of competence – knowledge and/or skill, as required – for the task at issue.

Expert system – The knowledge-base of clinical practice codified in cyberspace, for ready retrieval, as needed, in the course of practice [16].
Note: Development of clinical expert systems has now become feasible (due to theoretical developments), and it would provide for major advancement of quality-assurance as well as cost-containment in respect to clinical medicine [16].

*Exposure** – Subjection to (possible) effect(s) – noxious or salutary – of an environmental factor.
Note 1: A person is not 'exposed' to a factor that is a feature of his/her constitution or behavior. In reference to such factors the term should be understood to be a misnomer.

Note 2: Exposure may be considered in reference to a *point source* – a singular one (a particular infected person, a particular batch of a vaccine, a particular supply of food, etc.).

*Factor** – Concerning a person's status in respect to a particular sickness or illness, or a population's level of morbidity from a particular illness, a cause of it (having become what it is); also: a causal determinant of the probability of a health phenomenon (event or state, in an individual) or the level of a morbidity (in a population). (Examples: For the occurrence of hemorrhagic stroke, a moderately high blood-pressure, relative to a lower BP, is a factor; and BP per se, level unspecified, is a factor bearing on the rate of occurrence of hemorrhagic stroke.) (L. *facere*, 'do, make.')

Note: It is common, though quite questionable, in medical contexts to use the word 'factor' in reference to a merely descriptive – acausal – determinant. (Example: age as a 'factor' in . . .)

*False negative** – Concerning a diagnostic test, its negative result in the presence of the illness at issue (for diagnosis).

Note: Like 'false positive,' 'false negative' in its common meaning is a gross *misnomer*. Meant by 'false negative' should be a test result that is erroneous, specifically in the meaning of being falsely negative. (Example: in the pursuit of diagnosis about a latent case of lung cancer, the radiologist's failure to perceive, in CT images, a suspicious 'nodule' when such a pattern, as defined, actually is perceptible.) (Cf. 'False positive.')

*False positive** – Concerning a diagnostic test, its positive result in the absence of the illness at issue (for diagnosis).

Note: 'False positive' should mean a test result that is erroneous, specifically in the meaning of being falsely positive. (Example: When, in the pursuit of diagnosis about a latent case of lung cancer, a radiologist perceives a suspicious nodule, (s)he is producing a false-positive result [of the imaging test] if the 'lesion' actually is but a vessel's cross-section.) In its prevailing meaning the term, like 'false negative,' is a gross *misnomer*.

Fatality – In clinical medicine, death as the outcome of (the course of a case of) an illness.

*Fatality rate** (synonyms: case-fatality rate, death rate) – See 'Case-fatality rate.'

Finding – An abnormality or anomaly discovered in the process of investigating a client's state of health.

Good diagnosis/etiognosis/prognosis – One with probability close to that of correct diagnosis/etiognosis/prognosis.

Note: 'Good prognosis' is commonly attributed to an illness, as a common misnomer for not-so-bad course, 'bad prognosis' being its corresponding misnomer for bad course. However, prognosis actually is a cognitive entity, possible only for a doctor to have; as the illness of a doctor's patient does not have a mind, it cannot have prognosis. (Cf. Note 4 under 'Diagnosis.')

Gnosis – In medicine, a doctor's esoteric knowing about the health of a/the client; it encompasses diagnosis, etiognosis, and prognosis (descriptive pgn. and intervention-pgn.).

Note 1: This collective term for the three types of esoteric knowing that epitomize the learned professions of medicine is a recent neologism [16] – as also is 'etiognosis' as a member of this triad [25].

Note 2: The *knowing* in gnosis is about something hidden (as in science) but particularistic (different from science); and it may be wrong (as in science). By being particularistic, it does not qualify as knowledge (in the scholarly meaning of 'knowledge').

*Hazard** (synonym: health hazard) – A (potential) cause of illness, to be avoided, if possible.

*Health** – Concerning an individual at a given time, absence of ill-health/illness, overall or as for a particular type of illness (as in, say, 'cardiac health'); also: an individual's status in respect to presence/absence of a particular illness, or a population's level of morbidity from it, at a given time; also: the work of medical professions together with that of paramedical ones (cf. 'Community health' and 'Public health').

Note: It would be nice to have a term other than 'health' for that which in the individual context (time-specific) encompasses not only the absence of illness but also the presence of illness, just as, say, 'gender' – much better than 'man' or 'male' – denotes the person-characterizer whose categories are man/male and woman/female.

*Healthcare** (health care, health-care) – All that is done by health professionals, paramedical as well as medical, in respect to their clients' health (in a doctor's care starting from the pursuit of esoteric knowing about it). (See Note under 'Health services.')

*Health services** (synonym: healthcare) – See 'Healthcare.'

Note: 'Health services' actually is somewhat of a misnomer for healthcare at large. For, the broadest categories of healthcare, beyond the pursuit and attainment of gnosis (by doctors), actually are education, service, and regulation (incl. regulation of access to intervention, medicational or other); and while education might be viewed as being a service of sorts, regulation definitely isn't. (L. *servus*, 'slave.')

History – In the pursuit of gnosis in clinical medicine, the facts/factoids assembled from past records and/or client interview. (Cf. 'Anamnesis.')

Note: Under history in this meaning are subsumed also facts/factoids about *current* status as to symptoms (such as pain).

*Hygiene** (synonym: preventive medicine) – See 'Preventive medicine' under 'Medicine.'

*Iatrogenesis** – Concerning a sickness or an illness, etiogenesis by an action of a physician. (Gr. *iatros*, 'physician.')
      Note: Iatrogenesis of a sickness or an illness is not inherently a consequence of a medical error. For example, a particular type of sickness from a prescribed medication can be fully expected and accepted as such, and an idiosyncratic 'adverse drug reaction' is, in its first occurrence, not tantamount to an error of prescription. (Continued prescription would be an error).

*Idiosyncracy** – Reacting, or propensity to react, to a particular agent/stimulus in a manner that is quite peculiar to the individual at issue. (Gr. *idios*, 'own.')

*Illness** – Ill-health, specifically a somatic anomaly having at least the potential to become overtly manifest (in sickness; [10]). (Example: latent-stage cancer.) Principal subtypes:
      Defect (L. *vitium*) – Illness in which the defining somatic anomaly is a state. (Examples: vitium cordis, trisomy 21, various 'inborn errors of metabolism,' and various sequelae of diseases and injuries).
      Disease (L. *morbus*) – Illness in which the defining somatic anomaly is a process ('disease process') resulting from an intrinsic pathogenetic process (as in carcinogenesis, say; [11]). (Examples: morbus addisonii, communicable disease, and cancer.)
      Injury (Gr. *trauma*) – Illness in which the defining somatic anomaly is a process resulting from an extrinsic infliction (rather than from an intrinsic pathogenetic process; cf. 'Disease' above). (The outcome of injury commonly is a defect, as with, e.g., birth trauma.)
      Note: The I.E.A. dictionary [4] defines injury thus: "The transfer of one of the forms of physical energy (mechanical, chemical, thermal) in amounts or at rates that exceed the threshold of human tolerance. It may also result from lack of essential energy such as oxygen (e.g., drowning) or heat (e.g., hypothermia)." (A distinction is to be made between injury and etiogenesis of it: hypothermia, e.g., is not an injury, even if potentially injurious.)

*Impairment** – Worsening; also: the result of worsening.
      Note: The result of impairment can be a defect, but a defect need not be the result of a worsening (trisomy 21, e.g., isn't).

*Incidence** – Concerning an *event* of sickness/illness, its (pattern of) occurrence in a/the population being cared for (in community medicine), or among a clinician's clients, or in the abstract (in a particular category of people). (Cf. 'Prevalence.')

Note: The event at issue in what is thought of as the incidence of a chronic illness actually tends to be that of its first rule-in diagnosis.

Incidence rate* – See 'Rate.'

Indication – Concerning a particular somatic state, an available fact (or set of facts) pointing to its presence (possibly retrospective or prospective); also: concerning an intervention, a fact (or set of facts) about its potential recipient, making it an option to consider. (Cf. 'Contra-indicaton.')

Indicator – An aspect – a dimension – of something the realization of which gives an indication of something else. (Example: The result aspect of a diagnostic test serves as a diagnostic indicator, as it gives, by its particular realization, an indication of the presence/absence of the illness at issue.)
Note: Distinction-making in clinical medicine is based on diagnostic, etiognostic, and prognostic indicators. Prognostic indicators for adverse events/states are properly termed *risk indicators*; they need not be risk factors.

Indirect standardization* – See 'Rate' (Note 8).

Induction period* – The time lag from the inception of etiogenesis by a given factor to the resulting illness (its latent inception or an overt case of it). (Cf. 'Latency period.')

Injury* – See 'Illness.'

Intervention* – In clinical medicine, introduction/maintenance of a somatic artifact (presence of a medication, say) to enhance quality and/or quantity of life as they relate to sickness and illness, respectively; and in community medicine, introduction/maintenance of a program of communal change to reduce morbidity/mortality.
Note 1: An intervention is either *preventive/prophylactic*, or *therapeutic/palliative*, or *rehabilitative* in its intent. In clinical medicine it is any of these, as needed and feasible. In community medicine it generally is preventive (by regulatory change in people's environments or by service).
Note 2: The *application of a test* (gnostic) is not an intervention. For it doesn't change a person's soma and therefore does not, in itself, change the course of the person's health.
Note 3: A doctor's *teaching* a/the client how their health could be changed for the better is not an intervention either; for, like testing, it does not, in itself, change the course of health.
Note 4: Nor is a person's *change of 'lifestyle'* in response to a doctor's teaching/education an intervention. For, different from an intervention, it is not an artifact intended to change the natural course of health; it is, instead, a change in what makes for the natural course of health.
Note 5: One aim of community-level health-education is to be enhancement of people's knowledge about rational seeking of clinical interventions (latent-stage treatment of cancer, say).

Investigation – In medicine, the pursuit of gnosis; also: a testing or other fact-finding involved in this. (Examples: investigation of a pattern of occurrence for diagnosis about a possible epidemic; and investigation of a recognized epidemic as to its etiogenesis.) (Cf. 'Study.')

Knowledge-based medicine – Medicine that is genuinely professional; that is, medicine in which gnosis (this esoteric but particularistic knowing) is based on (general) medical knowledge (rather than being, notably, 'evidence-based' pseudo-gnosis, based on personal opinion about evidence [16]. (Cf. 'Evidence-Based Medicine' as well as 'Diagnosis,' 'Etiognosis,' and 'Prognosis.').

*Latency period** – The time lag from the inception of an illness (its definitional somatic anomaly) to the inception of its overt/clinical manifestation(s). (Cf. 'Induction period.')

*Latent** (antonyms: patent, overt, clinical) – Concerning a case of an illness (a cancer, say), the quality (transient, perhaps) of not being clinically manifest (in sickness).

Management – Concerning a case of a sickness or of an illness, the aggregate of actions (medical) to take care of it.

*Measurement** – A procedure to produce a result as a piece of information for the assessment of a magnitude of interest. (Example: sonographic measurement of left-ventricular ejection-fraction.) (Cf. 'Assessment.')
    Note: In assessing a client's health by taking a measurement of an aspect of it, the result of the measurement is not generally taken at 'face value' in respect to what is being measured, as allowance commonly needs to be made – judgmentally – for possible *error* in the result.

Medicine – A professional's pursuit and attainment of esoteric knowing about the health of the client – medical gnosis, that is – and teaching the client (or a representative of the client) accordingly. (Anything else – intervention, most notably – is incidental to, and not in the essence of, medicine; i.e., it is not always true of, and unique to, medicine. Cf. Preface and sect. I – 1. 1.)
    Clinical medicine – That segment of medicine in which individuals are cared for, one at a time. (Cf. sect. 1. 1.)
    *Community medicine** (synonym: epidemiology) – That segment of medicine in which 'communities' – populations (jurisdictional, occupational, ...) – are cared for as populations, rather than as individuals one at a time. (Cf. sect. I – 1. 1.)
    *Preventive medicine** – That segment of medicine which is directed to prevention of illness (from occurring).
    Note 1: Among epidemiologists there is a tendency to think that preventive medicine is subsumed, entirely, under community medicine (which in all essence is preventive medicine). But much of clinical medicine, too, is preventive. (Cf. 'Curative.')

Note 2: Epidemiologists like to think of prevention as also subsuming interventions on the course of illness – clinical interventions, that is. (Cf. 'Prevention' in sect. II – 2.)

Note 3: There is a tradition to distinguish between medicine and *surgery*, with the implication that surgical disciplines are not medical (but paramedical). It is to be understood, however, that a discipline ('specialty') of surgery is medical insofar as pursuit of gnosis and provision of gnosis-based 'doctoring' (teaching) are involved. The engagement in surgical interventions is no more antithetical to medicine than is, for example, the injection of medications in non-surgical medicine.

*Morbidity** – The (pattern of) occurrence of a particular illness in the cared-for population (quantified by the rate of this) in community medicine, or in the abstract (in a particular category of people). (See 'Comorbidity,' 'Incidence,' and 'Prevalence.')

Mortality – The (pattern of) occurrence of death, either from any cause or from a particular one, in the cared-for population (quantified by the rate of this) in community medicine, or in the abstract (in a particular category of people).

*Mortality rate** – The rate of occurrence of death, either from any cause or from a particular one, in the cared-for population in community medicine, or in the abstract (in a particular category of people). (Cf. 'Case-fatality rate' and 'Death rate.')

Note: All-cause rates of mortality are of express concern in *demography*. In community medicine, cause-specific rates of mortality – available as routine statistics – serve as useful indicators of what is the express concern: rates of *morbidity* from particular illnesses.

Natural course – Concerning an illness or sickness from it, the course of this in the absence of any treatment. (Cf. 'Natural history.')

*Natural history** (synonym: natural course) – See 'Natural course.'

Note: 'Natural history' is a still-common (bad) misnomer for natural course (of an illness). See 'Natural history' in section I – 2. 2. (Gr. *historia*, 'inquiry'; *histōr*, 'learned man.')

Negative – Concerning the result of a diagnostic test, the quality of not pointing to the presence of an illness. (Cf. 'Positive.')

*Normal** (antonym: abnormal) – Concerning an aspect of a person's soma at a particular time, whether structurally or functionally, or the result of a test to address this, the quality of being more-or-less usual for people of the same age (and gender, perhaps) in the same non-illness situation (at a given stage of pregnancy, or when finishing a marathon run, say).

*Nosocomial** – Pertaining to a hospital; also: concerning an illness, the quality of originating in a hospital. (Gr. *nosokomos*, 'person who tends the sick'; *nosos*, 'illness'; *komein*, 'to take care of.')

Nosology – Classification of illnesses. (Gr. *nosos*, 'illness.')

Noxiousness – The quality of being harmful to health. (L. *noxa*, 'injury, damage.')
(Cf. 'Safety.')

*Occurrence** – In clinical medicine, concerning an event of sickness/illness, its
taking place, and concerning a state of sickness/illness, its being present; and in
community medicine, the pattern of the individual occurrences of an event or a state
of sickness/illness. (Cf. 'Incidence' and 'Prevalence.')
   Note: A clinician's concern is a singular occurrence/non-occurrence in the individual client, while an epidemiologist's concern is the frequency – rate – of its
multiple occurrences in the client population, each at a given point in time or in
a given period of time.

*Outcome** – Concerning a disease or an injury, with its course not interrupted by
death from another cause, the end state of the process (fully restored health, a
sequela or a set of sequelae, or being dead from it); also: concerning an intervention, a/the result of it, in a given case, possibly causally but generally in descriptive,
acausal terms (as the effect generally cannot be inferred ad hoc).

Overdiagnosis – Rule-in diagnosis about a particular illness when that illness
actually is not present.
   Note: Recently, various critics of screening for a cancer have adduced a very
different concept of overdiagnosis: rule-in diagnosis about a latent, preclinical case
which never will become patent/overt/clinical on account of death from some other
cause. This represents the epitome of malformed concept.

Overt (synonyms: patent, clinical; antonym: latent) – Concerning a case of an
illness, the quality of (already) being manifest in sickness.

Palliation/palliative – Reducing sickness without ameliorating illness.

*Parameter** – In clinical medicine, any quantitative aspect/dimension of the client's
health, subject to measurement (by means of a test). (Example: systolic blood-
pressure.)

*Pathogenesis** – Concerning a disease or a defect (notably a sequela of a disease
or of an injury), the sequence of changes from normal structure and/or function to
the one definitional to the illness in question. It is a matter of how – rather than
why – an illness came/comes into being. (Example: in carcinogenesis, the sequence
of changes from normal tissue to neoplasia, through hyperplasia, dysplasia, and
metaplasia.) (Cf. 'Etiogenesis.')

Pathognomonic (synonym: diagnostic) – Concerning a symptom or a sign (possibly
from a laboratory test), or a cluster of these, the quality of being diagnostically

conclusive (i.e., justifying rule-in or rule-out dgn.). (Gr. *pathos*, 'illness'; *gnome*, 'a means of knowing').

Note: This is a generalization of the word's still-usual denotation, having to do only with a *clinical* sign, a *single* one in isolation, and limited to its quality of justifying *rule-in* diagnosis.

Patient – In clinical medicine, a physician's client in a given encounter with him/her, being cared for sickness or illness. (L. *patient*, 'suffering.')

Note 1: A physician's client seeking care on account of an abnormal result from a diagnostic test is analogous to one complaining about a symptom or a physical sign; (s)he is, in this encounter, a patient to the doctor.

Note 2: A client consulting a doctor about possible preventive care, or screening, is not the doctor's patient in this encounter, nor is a recipient of actual preventive care or of (the initial test in) screening.

Note 3: It remains commonplace among clinicians to think of all of their clients as patients of theirs, including between the encounters.

Note 4: In seeking access to clinical care, a doctor's client commonly has to be quite patient; and this could be taken to justify doctors' ubiquitous use of the term in reference to their clients.

Pattern recognition – See 'Diagnosis' (Note 2).

Physical examination – In the pursuit of gnosis in clinical medicine, ascertainment of current facts about the patient/client by means of the senses (incl. with their enhancement by means of auditory or visual aids).

*Physician** – A person authorized (licensed) to practice medicine.

*Point source** – See 'Exposure' (Note 2).

Positive – Concerning the result of a diagnostic test, the quality of pointing to the presence of an illness (commonly the illness at issue in the diagnosis). (Cf. 'Negative.')

*Positive (negative) predictive value** – Concerning positive (negative) result of a diagnostic test (in clinical medicine), the probability that this implies for the presence of the illness at issue.

Note: Both the term and the concept – common in 'clinical epidemiology' – are seriously *malformed*. At issue is not prediction (of the future) but knowing about the present; and diagnostic probability is determined by the entire diagnostic profile and not by a single test result in this [16]. It is very difficult to come up with an example of rational probability-setting for the presence of an illness in disregard for the person's age, for example.

Practice – Concerning healthcare, engagement in it; also: a clinician's particular office together with his/her engagement in healthcare.

Preclinical – Concerning a case of an illness or an illness in the abstract, the quality of it being in the latent stage of its development to an overt (clinical) case.

Prediction/predictive – See 'Positive (negative) predictive value' and 'Prognosis' (Note 4).

Prescription – A doctor's written instruction for the (preparation, dispensation, and/or) use of a medication (or for some other intervention).

*Prevalence** – Concerning a *state* of sickness/illness, its (pattern of) occurrence in a/the population being cared for (in community medicine), or among a clinician's clients, or in the abstract (in a particular category of people). (Cf. 'Incidence.')

Prevalence rate – See 'Rate.'

Prevention/preventive* – See 'Intervention' (Note 1).

*Preventive medicine** (synonym: hygiene) – See 'Medicine,' 'Curative,' and 'Intervention' (Note 1).

Primary diagnosis – Diagnosis related to, and explaining, the sickness/complaints of the patient. (Cf. 'Secondary diagnosis.')

Professionalism – Concerning a professional, the quality of functioning as well as reasonably is expected (of a professional).
  Note: In the present, science-related context, the salient feature of clinical professionalism is rejection of the anti-expert, subjectivist dilettantism of the EBM movement [16]. (See 'Evidence-based medicine' and 'Knowledge-based medicine.')

Profile – Concerning gnostic probability-setting, the set of available, relevant facts/factoids on the case.

Prognosing (synonym: prognosticating) – Pursuing prognosis; also: setting (specifying) prognosis (the probability of this) for a particular course or outcome.
  Note: 'Prognosing' as a synonym for 'prognosticating' is a here-proposed neologism, patterned after 'diagnosing.'

Prognosis – A doctor's esoteric knowing about the future course and/or outcome of a/the client's health, specifically in respect to a particular illness (cf. 'Diagnosis' and 'Etiognosis'):
  Clinical prognosis – A doctor's (clinician's) esoteric knowing about whether a particular, currently absent illness (overt) will occur; also: regarding an already-existing illness, such knowing (probabilistic) about an adverse event/state (treatment induced perhaps) in its course and/or as its outcome; also: a clinician's prognosis based on 'clinical' indicators alone (exclusive of laboratory test results).

Note 1: Whatever may be the possible prospective event or state at issue, *distinctions* generally are made in prognosis about it according to choice of intervention and period/point of prognostic time, as well as the prognostic profile at the time of the prognostication; and besides, a meaningful prognosis is conditional on surviving to the prospective time at issue.

Note 2: Clinical prognosis is knowing about the *correct probability* of the event's occurring or the state being present in/at a particular period/point of prognostic time. *Correct prognosis* is characterized by this probability, which represents the proportion of instances of the profile in general (in the abstract) such that, given the intervention, the event/state would occur in/at that period/point of prognostic time. (That proportion is implied by a suitable prognostic probability function.)

Note 3: An illness does not have a prognosis, good or bad (contrary to common parlance in clinical medicine); the doctor does. (Cf. 'Good diagnosis/etiognosis/prognosis.')

Note 4: Clinical prognosis generally is *not prediction*; it is prediction only when the set probability is very high (in absolute terms). Prognosis is knowing, while prediction need not be. Prediction is forecasting; and forecasting rain is giving a high probability for rain.

Community prognosis – A doctor's (epidemiologist's) esoteric knowing about the future course of the cared-for population's health, specifically about future levels of morbidity from a particular illness (in the population's recovery from an epidemic, say).

Note 5: Community prognosis, different from clinical prognosis, is prediction, forecasting (akin to forecasting weather).

Descriptive prognosis – Prognosis conditional on the choice of intervention.

Intervention prognosis – Prognosis about the effect(s) of an intervention; that is, the difference between the descriptive prognosis conditional on a particular intervention and its particular alternative.

Note 6: 'Descriptive' and 'intervention' prognosis are recently-proposed, novel terms (and concepts [16]).

Prophylaxis/prophylactic* – Reducing risk/rate of sickness or illness.

Public health* – Healthcare in the public domain, paramedical as well as medical; also: the 'public's' (the jurisdictional 'general population's') health (level of morbidity, generally in illness-specific terms).

Note 1: Before national health-insurance, the professional meaning of 'public health' was specifically that of community medicine (i.e., epidemiology) together with paramedical community-oriented healthcare (preventive); but upon the advent of national health-insurance, *clinical medicine* has come to trump community medicine as a public-health concern (as a matter, mainly, of quality-assurance and cost-containment, but of accessibility also).

Note 2: Quality-assurance in respect to clinical medicine requires quality-assessment of it, in the framework of national health-insurance by epidemiologists practicing public health. This practice could reasonably be termed *clinical epidemiology*. (Cf. Note 2 under 'Evaluation.')

Quasi-scientific medicine – Medicine that is like scientific medicine, except that the gnostic probability functions, GPFs, codify experts' tacit knowledge in lieu of scientific knowledge [16]. (Cf. 'Gnostic expert paneling' in sect. III – 4.)

Rate* – Concerning a sickness or an illness – an event (e.g., first rule-in diagnosis of a chronic illness) or a state (notably a chronic illness per se) – its frequency of occurrence in the population being cared for (in a community-medicine practice), or among the clients cared for in a clinical-medicine practice, or in the abstract.

Incidence rate* (particularistic, crude) – Concerning the occurrence of a particular type of health *event*, its frequency of occurrence in a particular amount of opportunity for its occurrence, specifically the number of these events occurring divided by the amount of opportunity for these events to occur.

Note 1: Only persons *at risk* for the phenomenon are legitimately seen to be contributory to the 'amount of opportunity' entering into a rate of incidence. (Cf. Note under 'At risk.')

Note 2: For a *proportion*-type rate of incidence (as with, e.g., the rate of adverse reactions to a vaccination, or the case-fatality rate for a particular illness), the 'amount of opportunity' is the number of instances in the referent of the rate (the number of vaccinations, say, or the number of cases of a particular illness cared for, say).

Note 3: For a rate of incidence in the meaning of incidence *density* (as with the rate of a cancer's incidence, in community medicine, in terms of the number of rule-in diagnoses [initial] divided by the amount of population-time for which the rate was documented), the 'amount of opportunity' is the amount of the population-time (commonly in person-year units) in the referent of the rate.

Note 4: When incidence density operates in a cohort-type population (sect. II – 4) for a particular period of time, this produces its corresponding *cumulative* rate of incidence, a proportion-type rate of incidence different from the type addressed above [12]. It is conditional on absence of intercurrent deaths (from extraneous causes, if at issue is death from a particular cause).

Prevalence rate (particularistic, crude) – Concerning the occurrence of a particular type of health *state*, its frequency of occurrence (presence) in a particular amount of opportunity for its occurrence, specifically the number of the instances (person-moments) in which it was/is present divided by the number of instances in which it (theoretically) could have been present; that is, the proportion of instances (person-moments) in the rate's referent such that the state at issue was/is present. (Cf. Note 1 above.)

Note 5: Rates (of incidence or prevalence) derived in this way are termed *crude* rates by epidemiologists; rates of this type are *overall* rates for their respective referents in the very terms that the experience presented itself – a given total number of the events/states occurred in a given total amount of opportunity for their recurrence. Given that the experience was heterogeneous in the sense of involving strata (by age and gender, say) of varying levels of typical risk for the event/state at issue, a crude rate reflects not only the stratum-specific rates but also the particular distribution of the experience across those strata. It inherently is the weighted average of those *specific* rates with weights proportional to the respective sizes of the stratum-specific experiences contributing to the crude overall rate.

Note 6: A crude overall rate commonly raises the question of what the overall rate (crude) would have been had the relative amounts of experience with the risk strata been different, in a particular way, from what they actually were, with the stratum-specific rates the same as they actually were/are. That different distribution (hypothetical, counterfactual) of the experience implies its corresponding weights for the stratum-specific rates and leads to the correspondingly *adjusted* overall rate.

Note 7: When two or more overall rates are compared with a concern for 'comparability' – freedom from influence of differential distributions across a particular set of strata of risk – the compared overall rates are adjusted to one-and-the-same – a shared – distribution (hypothetical). The resulting rates are said to be (mutually) *standardized* (in respect to distribution across the strata).

Note 8: It remains a common notion among epidemiologists that standardization in the meaning of invoking a shared set of weights (above) is but one possible 'method' of standardization – the *direct* standardization; and to this there is seen to be an alternative – *indirect* standardization. The misunderstanding in this has been exposed long ago [12] but it persists, including in the I.E.A. dictionary [4].

Note 9: A rate does not have a numerator and a denominator; it is the *result of dividing* the numerator input to its computation by the corresponding denominator input. (Cf. Preface.)

Note 10: The I.E.A. dictionary [4] declares, quite inexplicably and wholly without justification, that a proportion-type measure of frequency is not a rate. (Cf. Preface.)

Rehabilitation/rehabilitative – Enhancing adaptation to sequela(e) of illness.

Result – Concerning the application of a test (in clinical medicine), the datum or data produced by this (sans inference – gnostic – upon addition of the datum/data to the gnostic profile).

*Risk** – Concerning an adverse phenomenon (event or state) of health in the case of an individual, the probability (objective) that it will occur, given the prognostic profile of the person together with the choice of intervention (prospective); also: a health hazard.

Note: Risk in that first meaning is the *correct prognosis* in respect to the occurrence at issue. For the concept to be meaningful, needed is the same specificity and conditionality that characterizes meaningful prognosis. (See 'Prognosis.')

Rule-in diagnosis – Firm (high-probability) diagnosis affirming the presence of a particular illness (in a particular instance, in clinical medicine).

Rule-out diagnosis – Firm (high-probability) diagnosis affirming the absence of a particular illness (in a particular instance, in clinical medicine).

Safety – Concerning an intervention, the extent to which it is free of unintended, adverse effects. (Cf. 'Efficacy.')

Salubrious (synonym: salutary) – See 'Salutary.'

Salutary – The quality of being conducive to health. (L. *salus*, 'health.')

Scientific medicine – Medicine with a rational theoretical framework and knowledge-base from science [16, 19]. (Cf. 'Quasi-scientific medicine.')
  Note: Two conceptions of the role of science in the practice of medicine emerged in the 20th century [16]. One of these was imbedded in the famous and highly influential 'Flexner report' on medical education, published in 1910. The idea was that experience in the laboratories of the 'basic' medical sciences, in medical school, serves to develop, in the student, a scientific mind; and that the thus-developed scientific way of thinking is essential for successful problem-solving in the practice of medicine. Then, in 1992, a working group on 'evidence-based medicine' introduced a 'new paradigm,' in terms of which deference to experts' precepts was to be replaced by practitioners' individual critical readings of current literature on studies, original and derivative, and their taking this to be the basis of their respective practices. This idea, too, has turned out to be highly influential. Both doctrines are profoundly wrong-headed [16].

*Screening** – Pursuit of early (preclinical) detection of (i.e., of early rule-in diagnosis about) a particular illness.
  Note: The clinical concept of screening for an illness is the entire process/algorithm that may lead to early detection of the illness (but usually stops on account of negative result of the initial diagnostic test); but among epidemiologists the concept is, at present, confined to the initial test ("which can be applied rapidly" and may result in referral for further diagnostics in clinical care [4]).

Secondary diagnosis – Diagnosis unrelated to the sickness/complaints of the patient. (Cf. 'Primary diagnosis.')

*Sensitivity** – See 'Sensitivity and specificity.'

*Sensitivity and specificity** – Concerning a diagnostic test whose result is classified (unjustifiably, perhaps) as either positive or negative, the probabilities, respectively, of the positive result conditionally on the presence of the illness at issue and the negative result conditionally on the absence of the illness at issue.
  Note 1: One of the favorite topics of 'clinical epidemiologists,' advocating 'Evidence-Based Medicine,' these two quantities are falsely thought of as single-valued characteristics of the test in the application at issue [16]. In truth, the

distribution of a diagnostic test's result is prone to be highly dependent on the pre-test diagnostic profile [28].

Note 2: Both of these terms are misnomers for their referent concepts. Examples: A diagnostic test the result of which is a highly discriminating indicator of *risk* for the illness at issue is not 'sensitive' to actual presence of the illness; and any test from among the thousands that are available has, in these terms, a high 'specificity' to almost any illness!

Note 3: A diagnostician naturally wishes to have a diagnostic test that is 'sensitive' to the presence of the illness at issue; but (s)he should understand that the proper meaning of this is the test result's propensity to *change* (from normal to abnormal) in response to the presence of the illness. And (s)he naturally values specificity, too; but (s)he should understand that specificity really has to do not with a test per se but with a test *result*, its being specific (pathognomonic) to the presence or the absence of the illness at issue.

Note 4: Relevant to know about any diagnostic test, considered for a given type of application, is not its 'sensitivity' and 'specificity' in those meanings of the two but the prospects/probability, specific to the pre-test diagnostic profile, that the post-test diagnostic probability, corresponding to the test-augmented profile, would be practically 'conclusive' [16].

Sequela (plural: sequelae) – In clinical medicine, a defect as an/the outcome of the course of a disease or an injury. (Example: cirrhosis of the liver as the sequela of a case of hepatitis.)

Note: An illness is not causal – etiogenetic – to its sequelae; it is pathogenetic to them (Cf. 'Complication.')

*Sickness** (antonym: wellness) – Symptom(s) and/or overt sign(s) of illness (i.e., of a somatic anomaly), or unwellness from a cause other than an illness [29]. (A sick person can be perfectly healthy, only overcome by the circumstances – like an automobile, with nothing wrong with it, being unable to move when stuck in ice and snow.)

Note: Non-illness causes of sickness fall in the same general categories as do the causes of illness: constitutional (as in, e.g., 'morning sickness' in pregnancy), behavioral (as in, e.g., 'athlete's sickness' resulting from short but intense exertion), and environmental (as in, e.g., 'altitude sickness' resulting from low concentration of oxygen in high-altitude air).

Sign – Concerning an illness, a particular case of it or in general, an objective manifestation of it which, by its presence, is an indication of the presence of the illness.

Note: It remains commonplace to restrict the meaning of 'sign' to abnormal findings from physical examination (incl. clinical tests), that is, to overt – 'clinical' – abnormalities; but there is no good reason for not having the concept encompass abnormal results from laboratory tests as well.

Soma – The body (as distinct from the mind). (Gr. *sōma*, 'body.')

*Specificity** – See 'Sensitivity and specificity.'

Specific rate – See 'Rate' (Note 5).

*Standardized rate** – See 'Rate' (Notes 7 and 8).

Status – Concerning a person's soma, its state of being, in a particular regard at a particular time. (Examples: status post myocardial infarction; status asthmaticus.)

Study – In the pursuit of gnosis, a laboratory-type testing. (Examples: a radiographic 'study,' and a bacterial culture followed by 'study' of the organism's antibiotic sensitivity.) (Cf. 'Investigation.') (See 'Result.')

Subacute – Concerning a sickness or an illness, or an epidemic, the quality of being intermediate between acute and chronic.

Surgery – See 'Medicine' (Note 3).

*Survival rate** – The complement of case-fatality rate; also: the proportion of persons with a recognized case of an illness surviving a defined period of time or longer after the (initial) rule-in diagnosis. (See Note under 'Case-fatality rate.')

*Susceptibility** – The propensity to exhibit the effect, given the presence of a cause; also: concerning a sickness or an illness, being prone to come down with it.

Symptom – Concerning an illness, a particular case of it or the illness in general, an inherently subjective manifestation – overt, clinical – of it. (Prime example: pain.)

Symptomatology – The aggregate of symptoms.

*Syndrome** – A cluster of symptoms and/or signs taken to be definitional to a particular illness or pathognomonic for diagnosis about it. (Examples: Down's 'syndrome' as an illness, before its underlying anomaly was understood usually to be trisomy 21; and stroke 'syndrome' as pathognomonic of stroke.)

Test – In clinical medicine, a procedure potentially eliciting a sign of an illness. (See 'Sign' and 'Result.').
   Note: There are clinical as well as laboratory tests. (Examples: Aaron's test to potentially elicit a sign of appendicitis; glucose tolerance test to potentially elicit a sign of Type II diabetes.)

Therapeutic/therapy – Agent or action serving to ameliorate the course of an illness. (Cf. 'Palliation/palliative'; Gr. *therapeuein*, 'to medically administer.')

Treatment – Therapeutic or palliative action; also: intervention on the course of a (patho)physiologic risk factor.

Underlying cause – See 'Cause' (Note 2).

I – 2. TERMS AND CONCEPTS OF SCIENCE

I – 2. 1. Introduction

Epidemiological research, and clinical research just the same, is science in the original and still principal meaning of the word, namely that for which the term used to be 'natural philosophy' or 'natural history' (Gr. *historia*, 'inquiry'). Now the term generally is *natural science* – or, simply, *science*. This is the meaning of 'science' here. ('Science' entered the English language in the 19th century.)

The concept of science still is, principally, one of process, the activities of scientific inquiry, scientific *research*; but an added meaning of the word is the *knowledge* derived from the research. (Plato's and Aristotle's word for scientific knowledge was *epistēmē*.)

Scientific research on, and knowledge about, Nature has as its *objects* various *truths* about Nature, generally truths that are *abstract* – meaning abstract-general (placeless and timeless) rather than particularistic (spatio-temporally specific) – even if paleogeography and cosmology, for example, are in some respects exceptions to the concern, in science, only for abstract truths about Nature. (The reason for these exceptions is that the Earth and the cosmos have evolved, over enormous spans of time.)

The prevalence of malaria in a given place at a given time is not a potential object of epidemiological research (different from epidemiological practice concerned with that place at that time). The corresponding objects of epidemiological research and its resulting scientific knowledge are the ways in which malaria's rates of occurrence are in general – without reference to any particular place and/or time – functions of characterizers of people's constitutions, behaviors, and/or environments. There generally are no proper names (of places) in the objects of science, nor are there any references to calendar time (apart from some exceptions, noted above).

By the same token, the people participating in a 'trial' (experiment) on prophylaxis against malaria are not being studied in such a trial. The true object of the study is, in the main, the intervention's effectiveness in people in general, in the abstract, within the domain of the study (presence of potential indication for the intervention and absence of contra-indications for this, making distinctions among suitably

O. S. Miettinen, *Epidemiological Research: Terms and Concepts*,
DOI 10.1007/978-94-007-1171-6_2, © Springer Science+Business Media B.V. 2011

defined subdomains); and a secondary object is the intervention's safety, in equally 'universal' terms. The participating people are, simply, being exploited – upon their 'informed consent' – for the purpose of learning about something that in no way is specific to them.

Similarly, the 'study subjects' in an etiogenetic study are not being studied in the study: they contribute to a study of etiogenesis in an abstract domain.

Science (of Nature) is, already, differentiated into numerous separate, more-or-less independent *component sciences*, each with a relatively coherent overall *material object*, subject-matter. Thus, neuroscience – neurology in this meaning – is separate from, for example, cardiological science, from cardiology in this meaning (just as the corresponding disciplines of medicine are separate). The idea is that it is possible to study the neurological system – including illnesses of it – without broad and deep knowledge about the cardiovascular system, and vice versa.

Component sciences are not distinguished by their respective *formal objects,* nor by the methods they deploy. Thus, inquiry into the occurrence aspect of phenomena of health in humans does not constitute a science unto itself but is involved in many medical sciences (neuroscience, i.a.); nor does this epidemiological inquiry constitute or define a science even if it were to deploy (as has been commonplace to believe) 'the epidemiological method,' unique to this research.

Among particular sciences there are various shared methods of observation, methods of imaging between neurology and cardiology, for example. And there are, even, *shared methods of research, specific to shared types of formal object* of study, common across different sciences – shared methods for studying formal objects of the epidemiological and meta-epidemiological clinical types, for example. But, contrary to a common claim among philosophers, there is no general-purpose 'method of science' or 'scientific method,' applied in all of scientific research.

Instead of a common scientific method, by definition shared among all sciences is, for one, commitment to heed the imperatives of *logic* – and to deploy the faculty of *reason* more broadly – in the designs of the objects and methods of their studies, and in inferences (about the abstract objects of study) based on the results (particularistic) of the studies.

Also generally shared is the understanding that science is an intersubjective, *public* enterprise, and that this requires *objectivity* of communication about the objects, methods, and results of study. Statements about these should, as much as possible, have the same meaning for all concerned, in part by their sufficient *specificity* – and, apropos here, by the use of *appropriate terminology* to boot (cf. Introduction), now preferably in the lingua franca of modern science (English) first and foremost.

And as a science is about truths (about Nature, in natural science), the scientists' *truthfulness* about their work – and, equally, about the work of others, including about its perceived meaning for inference about the objects of study – is an overarching imperative in science. While science is central to the 'Baconian optimism' about progress in the human condition, Jacob Bronowski, in his venerable *The Ascent of Man* (1973), points out that those who have contributed to this ascent have been characterized by two qualities: "an immense integrity, and at least a little genius."

While "at least a little genius" characterizes the most consequential of scientists, "immense integrity" is expected of all of them.

I – 2. 2. Mini-dictionary

Where an asterisk (*) is here attached to a term, it indicates the term's inclusion in the I.E.A. dictionary of epidemiology [4].

Abstract (synonyms: general, abstract-general, universal; antonym: particularistic) – Concerning an object of inquiry and knowledge, the quality – generally definitional of science – of having a referent in neither place nor time; that is, being without a spatio-temporal referent; cf. sect. I – 2. 1 above.

Accuracy* – See 'Precision and accuracy.'

Analysis – See 'Analysis and synthesis.'

Analysis and synthesis – These two concepts are interrelated: "At the most elementary level, analysis concerns separation of a whole into its component parts, whereas synthesis is the reverse process of combining parts to form a complex whole" [30]. (Gr. *analuein*, 'unloose'; Gr. *syntheinai*, 'place together.')
   Note 1: Kant distinguished between analytic and synthetic judgments, calling them explicative and augmentative, respectively [31]. The former only analyze a conception as to its constituent conceptions, while the latter add to the conception a predicate which was not contained in it [31].
   Note 2: In their efforts to understand "the logical structure and empirical content of physical theory," subsequent philosophers have used the Kantian distinction (Note 1 above) extensively [30]. (Cf. 'Etiologic study' in sect. II – 4.)

Analytical* – See 'Analysis and synthesis.'

Applied* (antonym: pure) – Concerning a science, the quality of being application-oriented; that is, being intended to produce (by its research, potentially at least) knowledge of practical consequence. (Cf. 'Pure' and 'Basic versus applied research.')
   Note 1: The term and concept apply not only to segments of natural science and other empirical sciences but to parts of theoretical/formal sciences as well – statistics (as a branch of mathematics), for example.
   Note 2: Distinctions can be made between/among the degrees to which sciences, or topics within sciences, are 'applied.' Broadly, research in a 'basic' medical sciences is intended to potentially lead to an innovation for use in practices; but knowledge from quintessentially 'applied' medical research inherently provides for advancement of the very knowledge-base of practice [16].

Note 3: All of medical science, 'basic' medical science included, actually is 'applied' – supposed to have at least the potential to advance (the practice of) medicine. Research that deserves to be termed medical inherently is 'applied' [16].

Note 4: 'Applied' as a synonym for 'application-oriented,' while deeply and widely ingrained, is less than apposite. 'Instrumental' or 'practical' or 'pragmatic' might be better.

Applied research – See 'Basic versus applied research.'

Assumption – In theoretical sciences (such as mathematical statistics), a predicate taken as a given, without regard for whether it is true, to address what logically follows from it. (Cf. 'Presumption.')

Note: Assumptions are ubiquitous in theoretical (formal) sciences but have no place in empirical sciences.

Basic research – See 'Basic versus applied research.'

Basic versus applied research – As Peter Medawar (the Nobel laureate) in his *Pluto's Republic* (1982) disapprovingly put it, in medical academia the distinction is taken to be "between polite and rude learning, between the laudably useless and the vulgarly applied, the poetic and the mundane." (Cf. 'Applied,' Notes 2 and 3.)

Category (synonym: class) – A defined division in a system of classification. (See 'Nosology' in sect. I – 1. 2.)

Causality* – "The power or propensity that an object or event has to produce a change in itself or in another object or event" [32].

Note: "In the history of modern science, however, there has been no agreement about the concept, or even the existence, of causality" [32]. To Kant it was a "conception a priori," a "noumenon" in this meaning [31].

Concept – The abstract essence of a thing (entity, quality, relation), true of each instance of the thing and unique to it [1].

Note: A concept is specified by its *definition*, which, ideally at least, specifies the concept's proximate genus and its specific difference within this genus [1]. Examples: triangle is polygon (proximate genus) with three sides (specific difference); man is rational animal (Kant).

Conception – The formation of a concept; also: a concept.

Conclusion – The result of deductive reasoning.

Note 1: A conclusion is *formally correct* if the logic in the deduction is correct. It is also materially correct and hence *totally correct* only if, in addition, the two premises in the syllogism (the major and minor premise) are (materially) correct. (Cf. 'Proof.')

Note 2: In empirical science there is *no justifiable place* for inductive 'conclusions' such as are now commonly required (by journal editors) in the Abstract or Summary of each research report. (Cf. 'Induction' and 'Inference.')

Note 3: Useful *deductive* conclusions *are* possible in empirical science. Example: If it has been established that (a given type of) screening provides for earlier treatment of a cancer, and that earlier treatment of the cancer is more commonly life-saving than later treatment, it follows (as a matter of deductive logic) that (the particular type of) screening for the cancer provides for saving of lives (through earlier treatment).

Note 4: Remarkably, however, the prevailing governmental doctrines about 'outcomes research' in the U.S. (see sect. III – 2) are decidedly averse to such reasoning, insisting on the need for randomized trials to test the hypothesis about mortality-reduction (despite the enormous cost and other drawbacks of these trials; see 'RCTism' in sect. III – 4).

Corroboration – Successful reproduction of previous evidence. (Similar result from a similar study, apart from efficiency and/or size, perhaps.)

*Data** (plural of datum) – A body of recorded observations, directly empirical (and hence particularistic) facts or factoids. (See 'Observation.')

Datum – See 'Data.'

*Deduction** (synonym: deductive inference) – Reasoning from two givens (the major and minor premises) to a conclusion.

Note: The conclusion follows because the minor premise is a special case of the more general, major premise. (Cf. Note 3 under 'Conclusion'; in it, the major premise follows the minor one.)

Definition – See 'Concept.'

Derivative study – See 'Study' (Note 2).

*Design** – Concerning a study, the way it is structured; also: the way this structure, with empirical content, is brought about. (Examples: factorial design/structure; and bringing about the factorial structure by means of separate, independent randomizations, together with the way of making observations in this framework.) (See Notes under 'Analysis and synthesis.')

*Determinant** – When one quantity (a rate, say) depends on something else (causally or acausally), the latter is said to be a determinant of the former. (Example: The rate of incidence of a cancer generally depends on the population's distribution by age; that is, age generally is a determinant of the age-specific rate, its magnitude.) (Cf. 'Determinism.')

Note: A binary, 'all-or-none' outcome – the 'all' – is not a quantity, and it thus does not have determinants (while the probability/risk of this does have).

*Determinism** – The philosophical doctrine that every phenomenon of Nature, and every human action and cogitation likewise, is an inevitable consequence of its antecedents.

Note 1: As a story goes, a youngster had just been chided by a parent of his/hers about bad behavior; and (s)he, looking up to the parent, asked: do you think this is genetic, or perhaps only environmental?

Note 2: In these terms, even very serious wrongheadedness in science [33] is not something that the scientists themselves are accountable for.

*Dimension** – An aspect in which an object may be characterized; also: the non-numerical aspect of a dimension in this meaning. (Examples: concerning an illness, the incidence and prevalence dimensions of its occurrence; the inverse-time dimension of an incidence-density of its inceptions; and the dimensionlessness of a rate of its prevalence.)

Discovery – The attainment of a qualitatively new piece of knowledge about Nature, especially if based on a single study (which is exceptional). (Example: Jenner's epochal discovery – and demonstration – of the preventability of smallpox by means of vaccination with matter from blisters of cowpox.)

*Empirical** (antonyms: theoretical, formal) – Concerning a science, or a result of a study, or a belief, the quality of being based on experience – scientific, with its attendant reasoning – rather than on reasoning alone. (Cf. 'Empiricism.')

Empiricism – The epistemological doctrine of 'logical positivists/empiricists,' most notably in the Vienna Circle, who held that, as knowledge is justified only by experience, the truths of science are not necessary but only contingent, and that knowledge could not extend beyond experience [34]. (Cf. 'Nominalism,' 'Realism,' and 'Rationalism.')

*Epistemic** (synonym: epistemological) – See 'Epistemological.'

Epistemological (synonym: epistemic) – Concerning a topic in the theory of a science, the quality of having to do with methods of inquiry (about the abstract), the conceptual approaches in this (as distinct from, notably, instrumentation or other procedural aspects of research). (Cf. 'Ontological.')

Note: This is a proposed adaptation, to science, of the corresponding central concept in philosophy, in which epistemology is the study of knowledge (as to its nature, extent, and justification). (Gr. *epistēmē*, 'knowledge.')

*Epistemology** – See 'Epistemological' (Note).

*Evidence** – Concerning a study in empirical science, the product of it; that is, a study's reported result(s) together with the documented genesis of the result(s) – the genesis being the methodology of the study, as designed and, more importantly, as this design got to be implemented (incl. as a matter of deviations from the design).

Note 1: For more on evidence, see 'Study' and 'Result.'
Note 2: The result's genesis determines its qualities in respect to its degrees of *validity* and *precision*.

*Experiment** (antonym: non-experimental study) – See 'Observation and experiment.'

Explanandum (plural: explananda) – Something explained (potentially at least, by an explanans).

Explanans (plural: explanantia) – Something offered, or serving, as an explanation of something else, of an explanandum, that is. (Examples: The occurrence of an illness has its etiogenesis as a partial explanans; and the correct diagnostic probability conditional on a particular diagnostic profile would have the corresponding probability function as an explanans [16].)

Explanation – Concerning something known or presumed to be true, something else, also known or presumed to be true, that serves to remove the mystery in this, partially at least – by bringing the explanandum, to some extent at least, into the realm of the otherwise known. (Example: The known effect of the use of aspirin in reducing the risk of myocardial infarction has an explanation, partial, in the known effect of aspirin in reducing the adhesiveness and, hence, the aggregation of blood platelets.)

*Explanatory** – The quality of serving to provide an explanation, partial at least.

Fact – An objective observation (which presumably would have been agreed upon by all potential, qualified observers; cf. 'Objective'); also: a well-established piece of knowledge (possibly erroneous; cf. 'Knowledge').

Factoid – A semblance of a fact; that is, something that appears to be a fact, or is presented as a fact, but is nevertheless false.

*Factorial design** – Concerning two (or more) co-determinants in a study, design arrangement such that the distribution of one of them is the same at all levels, or in all categories, of the other(s), and conversely.

Finding – Coming, empirically, to an abstract 'truth' about Nature, presumptively at least, either 'finding' a hypothesis (or a theory's implication) to be 'true' or coming upon an unheralded, more-or-less serendipitous discovery; also: such a 'truth' per se. (Examples: based on measurement values for the degree of the bending of the paths of light beams in the gravitational field of the Sun, 'finding' an implication of Einstein's General Theory of Relativity to be 'true'; and 'finding' – discovering – H. Pylori to be the critical agent in the etiogenesis of peptic ulcer; also: the results of these 'findings.')

Note 1: A study result per se, without that inferential impact, is not a finding (of something qualitatively new, about Nature, in the abstract). This accords with the concept of finding in medicine (sect. I – 1.2).

Note 2: On a given topic in science there cannot be mutually discrepant findings, only discordance of evidence.

General (synonyms: abstract, abstract-general, universal) – See 'Abstract.'

*Generalization** – Concerning scientific knowledge, its extrapolation: given that something is known for a particular domain (a given gender of humans or a particular species of rodents, say), by inductive inference from experience specifically with this domain, taking this to mean that it thereby is also known or knowable – to some extent at least – for another domain (the other gender of humans or another species, say).

Note: In science one does not generalize from a 'sample' to a 'target population,' nor really from the particularistic to the abstract: the particularistic provides for *inference* about rather than generalization to – much less a conclusion about – the abstract. And as for etiogenetic research in particular, causation in the study experience is not an available fact (for generalization beyond this experience); it, already, would be an object of inference, but the real issue is inference about the abstract in the face of the available evidence. (Cf. 'Inference' and 'Conclusion.')

Genus (plural: genera) – A taxonomic category. (Example: disease as a genus of illness; cf. sect. I – 1. 2.)

Note: Genus is a subcategory of a taxonomic *family*, and a subcategory of a genus is a *species* of it. Example: communicable disease as a species of the genus disease in the family of illness.

Hermeneutics – The art of interpretation (originally of Scripture). (See 'Interpretation.')

*Hypothesis** – An idea in the meaning of a tentative piece of new (abstract) knowledge.

Note 1: A hypothesis – hypo-*thesis* – is more than a mere possibility, while remaining short of the status of knowledge. There is some reason to cautiously entertain the idea (according to those who do).

Note 2: Denial of a hypothesis is not a hypothesis ('null hypothesis'). It is, instead the stance expected of a scientist so long as there is no good reason to believe the hypothesis.

*Induction** (synonym: inductive inference) – The process of reasoning from a given but limited to something more general. (Example: reasoning from evidence – particularistic – to a state of Nature – abstract-general.) (Cf. 'Study,' Notes 3 and 4.)

Note 1: Different from deduction, induction *does not allow conclusion*. Arguably at least, inductive logic is a contradiction-in-terms.

Note 2: Knowledge in an empirical science is inductive and, therefore, fallible/uncertain. It is particularly uncertain in respect to causality, as this is not a phenomenon (but only a noumenon; cf. 'Causality').

*Inference** – Induction and/or deduction. See also 'Generalization,' 'Induction,' 'Result,' and 'Study' (Notes 2 and 4).

*Information** – Fact(s) documented and/or communicated.

Instrumental (synonym: applied) – See 'Applied.'

Interpretation – Concerning an evidentiary report, deciphering the meaning of it – what the evidence actually is (as a basis for inference about the object of study); also: concerning information more generally, deciphering what the information actually is. (Cf. 'Induction' and 'Inference.')
Note: Interpretation has to do with reception of a message. While a research report is a message, scientific evidence in a research report is not a message – from Nature to scientists. For, Nature is secretive rather than communicative about its truths.

*Interval scale** – See 'Scale' (Note 2).

Knowledge – Experts' consensus belief (possibly wrong) as to what an abstract truth is. (Gr. *epistēmē* is knowledge in this abstract-general meaning; cf. 'Gnosis.')
Note 1: From the vantage of an individual, a distinction is to be made between knowing something abstract and knowing *of* something abstract. When knowing something, one can justify one's sharing of the consensus belief of experts; otherwise the belief is but a *received* one, a matter of knowing *of* the consensus belief of experts. (In medicine, doctors generally do not know, e.g., the effects of the medications they prescribe; they only know *of* these.)
Note 2: Scientific knowledge is not the product of research per se. See 'Evidence,' 'Induction,' and Note 3 under 'Study.'
Note 3: Subjective knowledge is a contradiction-in-terms; it is but a subjective belief, rather a generally shared and in this sense an objective belief (which knowledge is).

Law – A formally (mathematically) expressed and well-established pattern of interrelation between phenomena. (Examples: Newton's laws of motion; laws of thermodynamics; and Ohm's law concerning electricity.)
Note: The double-helix structure of the DNA molecule is not a law of Nature, nor is the magnitude of Planck's constant; and while an empirical risk function for an illness is of the form of a law of Nature, it really is but descriptive of experience rather than of Nature in the abstract. Genuine laws of Nature are largely based on theoretical insights, confirmed by evidence.

Lemma – In a proof, a relevant subsidiary statement, taken to be true. (Example: In Note 1 under 'Conclusion' above, the deduction involves two lemmas.)

Lingua franca – A language used (as a medium of communication) among persons of diverse native languages.

Note: The lingua franca of *scientists* used to be Latin; now it is English.

Logic – The "science and art of correct thinking" [1].

Note: A formal distinction is to be made between *formal* and *material* logic (as Aristotle – the father of formal logic [among many other lines of scholarship] – already did). Formal logic is about reasoning per se, with no reference to subject-matter, whereas material logic (as in science) has both elements. *Theory of epidemiological research* – as for its terms and concepts and, especially, its principles – is a genre of material logic. Terms are included in this, as reason ultimately is the judge of what the admissible, tenable terms for the admissible, relevant concepts are.

*Measurement** – Concerning a presumed constant of Nature (the normal core temperature of the human body, say) or some particularistic quantity (a particular person's core temperature at a particular moment, say), a process producing an empirical value serving as an information input to quantification (inferential) of it, to assessment/estimation of the magnitude.

Note 1: In a study, measurement is production of an observation on a quantitative (interval or ratio) scale.

Note 2: Whereas observation on a purely qualitative (nominal) or ordinal (semi-quantitative) scale is not a result of measurement, errors of observation on such scales are not ones of wanting *precision* or wanting *accuracy*. They are, instead, matters of *misclassification*. (Cf. 'Precision and accuracy.')

*Misclassification** – Concerning an observation on a nominal or ordinal scale, classification of it in a category in which it does not belong. (Cf. Note 2 under 'Measurement.')

*Natural experiment** – A study in which the setting (for observations) is similar (or identical) in comparison with what in principle might be experimentally arranged, but this setting is a naturally occurring one rather than the result of selective assembly (as in a quasi-experiment) or artificial arrangement (as in an experiment).

Note 1: The term 'natural experiment' implies that an experiment can occur naturally, that the setting for experimental observations need not be artificial. But that is a contradiction-in-terms. Thus, 'natural experiment' is a self-contradictory term, a misnomer. The corresponding apposite term would be *natural quasi-experiment*.

Note 2: An example of a quasi-experiment in which the setting for observations is *not* naturally occurring is a non-experimental intervention study in medical research, one in which the study subjects with the contrasted interventions are assembled from some source population-time and the interventions are 'natural' in the meaning of not having been artificially arranged for the purpose(s) of the study.

*Natural history** – An archaic term for natural science. (Cf. sect. I – 1. 2.)

Natural quasi-experiment – See Notes under 'Natural experiment' (Note 1).

Natural science (synonym: science) – See 'Science.'

*Negative** – See Note 4 under 'Result.'

Nominalism – The philosophical doctrine that concepts (abstract) and judgments based on these have no objective referent but exist only in names (i.e., in terms and their purported interrelations). (Cf. 'Realism.')
    Note: In a discussion with me, very long ago, D.L. Sackett declared himself a nominalist and, thereby, unconcerned with what I view as malformed concepts in medicine. (At issue were a diagnostic test's 'sensitivity' and 'specificity.')

*Nominal scale** – See 'Scale' (Note 1).

*Non-experimental** (synonym: observational; antonym: experimental) – See 'Observation and experiment.' (Notes 1 and 2).

Noumenon – A thing (entity, quality/quantity, relation) that is not subject to sensory perception/observation but is, instead, a 'conception a priori' of the mind (Kant [31]). (Prime example: causation.) (Gr. *noumenon*, 'concept, thought.')

*Objective** – Concerning a purported fact (denotation of a term, or a datum's relation to the corresponding fact/truth, say), the quality of being agreeable by all potential, qualified judges.

Observation – The acquisition of a datum (empirical). See 'Observation and experiment.'
    Note: The 'observation' to which a research datum refers need not have been actually observed by the investigators. Thus, in an epidemiological study, a given number of deaths may have been 'observed' without any of the investigators actually having witnessed any of them to take place.

*Observational** (synonym: non-experimental; antonym: experimental) – Concerning a study (empirical), the quality of documenting what occurs naturally – in natural conditions, as distinct from artificial conditions arranged for the purposes of the study. (Cf. 'Observation and experiment.')
    Note 1: All experiments (with their artificial arrangements) also are observational in the meaning of involving observations (as does all empirical research). Thus, actually meant by 'observational study' is study that is *purely* observational (i.e., devoid of experimental arrangements/artifacts for the phenomena to take place and to be observed); meant is *non-experimental* study.
    Note 2: the observations in a scientific study generally do not take place naturally; artificial arrangements generally need to be made for these (Cf. 'Observation.')

*Observation and experiment** – The two foundations of knowledge in empirical sciences [35].

Note 1: That pair of terms for the conceptual duality, while traditional and still well-established, is less than apposite. The duality really is that constituted by *non-experimental* and experimental studies, both of these being 'observational' in the meaning of accruing observational facts – particularistic, directly or indirectly sensory – for the purpose of learning about something non-particularistic, something general in the meaning of abstract-general. (Cf. Note under 'Observational.')

Note 2: In non-experimental research, phenomena are observed in naturally occurring settings, though selectively and with forethought, and commonly with artificial arrangements for the observations themselves. The first corroboration of the General Theory of Relativity, concerning the bending of the paths of rays of light in a gravitational field, was *non-experimental*, as the light was issued by stars (during the solar eclipse of 1919). By contrast, the epoch-making Michelson-Morley study (in 1881, to study whether all-pervasive, stationary 'ether' actually exists), was *experimental* because the investigators themselves issued the light beams for the purposes of the study (to learn whether their speeds depend on their directions relative to the direction of the Earth's movement in space).

Note 3: Research on a diagnostic probability function is not experimental on the basis that artificial arrangements need to be made to observe – determine – the fact about the presence/absence of the illness at issue (cf. Note 1 above). But it is experimental if some of the diagnostic indicators are based on artificial arrangements for the study – experimental (rather than practice-based) radiography, for example.

*Occam's razor** – See 'Ockham's razor.'

Ockham's razor (synonyms: Occam's razor, principle of parsimony) – The ontological principle (ascribed to William of Ockham, not Occam) that the adopted set of concepts should be kept to the minimum necessary.

Note: Analogously, the *terms* denoting an adopted concept should be kept to the minimum necessary (commonly only one in any given language).

Ontal/ontic (synonym: ontological) – See 'Ontological.'

Ontological – Concerning a topic in the theory of science, the quality of having to do with the nature of the objects of inquiry and of the corresponding knowledge (about the abstract), especially as to their admissibility into the status of being legitimate objects of scientific inquiry and knowledge. (Example: The broadest and most fundamental ontic question for the development of the knowledge-base for scientific clinical medicine is about the generic nature – the form – of this knowledge; and the answer is: gnostic probability functions [16].) (Cf. 'Epistemological.')

Note: This is an adaptation, to science, of the corresponding central concept in philosophy, in which ontology is the study of the nature of being.

*Ontology** – See 'Ontological' (Note).

*Ordinal scale** – See 'Scale' (Note 1).

Original study – See 'Study' (Note 2).

Parsimony – In ontology, admitting only the minimum necessary set of concepts. (Cf. 'Ockham's razor.') (L. *parsus*, 'to spare.')
Note: Parsimony as a general virtue in science is distinct from a related other virtue: *simplicity* – giving preference to the simplest formulation or explanation among otherwise interchangeable ones. (Prime example: preference for the Keplerian astronomy over Ptolemy's.)

Phenomenon – A thing (entity, quality, relation) subject to sensory perception/observation (indirectly at least). (Examples: a genotype, an illness, a tumor's doubling time, and the prevalence of a state of health.) (Cf. 'Noumenon.')

Positive – See 'Positive study' in section II – 4.

*Precision** and accuracy** – Concerning measurement (for assessment of the magnitude of a parameter of Nature), the respective referent concepts of these terms are [36]:
Precision (synonym: reproducibility) – The degree of agreement among a set of observations – results of measurement of a parameter of Nature – after all known sources of error are accounted for.
Accuracy – The degree of agreement between the precise measure and the corresponding true magnitude (unknown).
Note 1: These definitions emerged following the publication of the method of least squares by C.F. Gauss in 1809 and 1823, and they've remained rather stable ever since [36].
Note 2: 'The precise measure' can be the one from an infinite number of hypothetical replications of a study. Accuracy in this meaning is freedom from *bias*.
Note 3: The prevailing terminology in epidemiology is at variance with this; see 'Accuracy,' 'Precision,' and 'Validity' in section II – 4.

Presumption – A predicate judged to be true. (Cf. 'Assumption.')
Note: In statistical science, statistical models represent presumptions, not assumptions.

Principle – Concerning a line of research (epidemiological or meta-epidemiological clinical, say), a dictate of logic (about correct thinking, especially in the designs of the objects and methods of study, but in the inferences also).

Principle of parsimony (synonym: Occam's/Ockham's razor) – See 'Ockham's razor.'

Proof – Concerning a proposition or a thesis, incontrovertible demonstration of its correctness.

Note: It has become quite generally agreed that proofs are unattainable in empirical sciences [37]. Their justified place is only in theoretical/formal sciences, in which ideas generally are subject proof as to truth/untruth, on the basis of reasoning alone. (Cf. 'Conclusion' and 'Lemma.')

Proposition – A statement expressing a tentative judgment, put forward for critical consideration by others.

Pure (antonym: applied) – Concerning a science, or a region within a science, the quality of the inquiries in it not being intended to be of any practical consequence. (Cf. 'Applied.')

*Quasi-experiment** – A study (scientific, empirical) in which the setting for observations is similar or identical in comparison with what might be experimentally arranged, but the setting actually is a non-experimental one – naturally occurring (cf. 'Natural experiment') or the result of selective assembly of the observables. As the term implies, quasi-experiment is like an experiment without actually being one (as for the genesis of the setting for the observations).

*Ratio scale** – See 'Scale' (Note 2).

Rationalism – The epistemological doctrine according to which at least some knowledge about Nature is justifiable without reference to experience [34]. (Cf. 'Empiricism.')

Note: To a rationalist, genuine knowledge (abstract) about Nature is not necessarily 'evidence-based.' (Cf. 'Thought experiment.')

Realism – The philosophical doctrine (opposite of nominalism) that the abstract – its concepts and the relations of these – is more real than the phenomenal (sensory) counterpart(s) of the abstract. (Cf. 'Nominalism.')

Note: Plato and Aristotle were realists; and realism is, implicitly, the philosophical basis for a dictionary (such as this one) on terms and *concepts* of a line of research.

Received knowledge – See Note 1 under 'Knowledge.'

*Replication** – Concerning a study, its repetition in the same way (apart from place and time, and study efficiency and size, perhaps) on the same object (scientific, inherently unchanging from a study to its repetition).

Note: Replication need not – and commonly does not – reproduce the previous result(s). It is the (at least potential) irreproducibility of a result that justifies – and commonly calls for – replication of an initial study on the object of study.

*Reproducibility** (synonym: precision) – See 'Precision and accuracy.'

*Research** – In natural science, inquiry into an abstract truth about Nature, specifically the studies on a given object of inquiry in the aggregate, as a whole. (Cf. 'Study.')

Note: Given the abstract nature of the objects of scientific inquiries (with some exceptions; see sect. I – 2. 1), any given object of scientific inquiry can be – and commonly needs to be – studied repeatedly (and as a practical matter, in different places at different times) – as *re*-search, *replicating* previous studies on it. (See 'Replication.')

Result – Concerning a piece of research, an/the essential datum – empirical counterpart of something theoretical that is descriptive of Nature – produced by it. (Example: the results on – the empirical values for – for the speed of light obtained in the epochal Michelson-Morley experiment.)

Note 1: Result of a piece of research in this meaning is analogous to any result produced by a diagnostic test/'study' (inquiry into the health of a patient): it is the *object-descriptive datum*, however imprecise and/or biased. A measure of imprecision (the datum's standard error, say) is not descriptive of the object of study (but, instead, of the study on the object of study).

Note 2: There are *no results on causality/effects*, as causation is not a phenomenon (subject to documentation in data). In research on causality the aim is to produce a result – inherently descriptive – for use in inference about causality.

*Scale** – Concerning a particular dimension of an object per se or of observations on it (temperature or gender, say), the terms of specifying its possible realizations (e.g., the Celcius scale, or the Kelvin scale, for temperature; and the male-female duality for gender).

Note 1: Among non-quantitative scales, a distinction is made between *nominal** and *ordinal** scales. The categories of a (strictly) nominal scale (that of gender, say) have no intrinsic ordering, different from the categories of an ordinal scale (that constituted by the successive stages in the pathogenesis, or progression, of a cancer, or the categories of severity for cases of a congenital heart-defect, say). An ordinal scale can be thought of as being semi-quantitative.

Note 2: Among quantitative scales, a distinction is made between *interval** and *ratio** scales. An interval scale has an arbitrary point for zero units (as has, e.g., the Celsius scale for temperature), whereas a ratio scale is one in which zero units coincides with nothingness as the magnitude of the object of the quantification (as is the case with the Kelvin scale for temperature: 0 °K is the temperature in which all molecules are completely motionless). An interval scale admits statements about differences between values (e.g., that 27 °C is 27 °C higher than 0 °C) but not about ratios of values (e.g., that 27 °C is an infinite multiple of 0 °C). By contrast, a ratio scale does admit ratio statements as well (e.g., that 300 °K [27 °C] is 10% higher than 273 °K [0 °C]).

*Science** (synonym here: natural science) – Inquiry (by research and induction based on its results) into abstract truths about Nature; also: the knowledge (abstract) about Nature derived by the inquiry.

Note: More on the essence of science sect. I – 2. 1, in Part II and Part III, and here under 'Study,' 'Result,' and 'Induction.'

*Serendipitous** – Concerning a discovery, the quality of having been achieved without a designed, methodical inquiry; that is, achieved by the application of acute intellection to an incidental observation. (Examples: discoveries of X-rays and penicillin.)

Simplicity – See Note under 'Parsimony.'

Study – A piece of research; that is, a project to produce evidence (for inductive judgments) about the abstract truth (unknown) at issue. (See 'Evidence,' 'Result,' and 'Induction.')
    Note 1: Inductive inference from the evidence produced by any given study may not be a proper concern in the context of the very first study on a given object of study. In this context the need may be for replication of the study before any inference (inductive) about the state of Nature.
    Note 2: Once the first study on a given object of research has been replicated by at least one other *original* study, the aggregate of available evidence – in statistical science, notably – generally is to be subjected to a *derivative* study, in which the evidence from all of the original studies is synthesized (critically).
    Note 3: In the face of the available entirety of evidence (commonly from derivative research), the need is for the translation of the evidence – through induction – into (updated) belief about the object of study. This is a task for members of the relevant *scientific community*, not for the researchers involved in the production of the evidence. (Those investigators are biased on the topic at issue, having a vested interest.)
    Note 4: While science translates evidence into knowledge (Note 3 above), science does not translate knowledge into (knowledge-based) choice of *action*. "Science never tells a man how he should act; it merely shows how a man must act if he wants to attain definite ends" [38]. "The role of a scientist is not to determine which risks are worth taking, or deciding what choices we should take, but . . . to determine what the possibilities are" [39].

Syllogism – Statement of a deduction (of a conclusion from its premises).

Synthesis – See 'Analysis and synthesis.'

*Taxonomy** – A system of classification. (Gr. *taxis*, 'arrangement, order.') (See 'Genus,' and also 'Nosology' in sect. I – 1.2.)

Test – Concerning a hypothesis, a study intended to provide evidence that either supports or takes away from the hypothesis; that is, either increases (by being positive) or decreases (by being negative) the credibility/plausibility of the hypothesis. (Cf. 'Positive' and 'Negative.')

Note: When the hypothesis implies the entire range of non-null values of the parameter being studied ('semi-infinite' in one direction, as is common in epidemiological research on etiogenesis of illness), a test result that is quite imprecise may be neither positive nor negative; the study may be quite uninformative, a failure except as a small contribution to a later derivative study.

Theorem – An idea that is demonstrably correct; that is, a proposition proven to be true. (Examples: Bayes' theorem and Central Limit Theorem, in probability theory and statistics, respectively.)

Note: There are no theorems in empirical science, only in theoretical/formal science. (Cf. 'Proof.')

Theoretical (antonym: empirical) – Concerning a science, the quality of its knowledge inherently being solely reasoning-based (as is true, most notably, of mathematics); also: concerning the magnitude of a quantity of Nature, its true but unknown value (as distinct from any empirical counterpart of this).

Theory – A grand and quite well supported thesis (no longer a mere hypothesis on its grand scale, but not yet knowledge either). (Examples: Darwin's idea about the evolution of species, and Einstein's general relativity, were theories rather than established truths before their general acceptances by the respective scientific communities.)

Thesis – A relatively forceful proposition, one that is advanced with considerable seriousness (as to belief in its correctness).

Thought experiment (synonym: Kantian experiment) – Imaginary experiment, to support/justify (or refute) an idea.

Note: Thought experiments were eminent in Einstein's physics.

Truth – In empirical science, the actual (hidden) way Nature is in a particular respect (this 'state of Nature' constituting an object of scientific inquiry).

Universal (synonyms: abstract, general, abstract-general) – See 'Abstract.'

I – 3. TERMS AND CONCEPTS OF STATISTICS

I – 3. 1. Introduction

One of the meanings of 'statistics' relates to affairs of the state (hence the term) or some other jurisdiction, and in this sense it is the art of the acquisition and presentation of aggregate data on the population, usually tabular in form. Statistics in this meaning has to do with census data, vital statistics (on births and deaths), and cancer-registry data, for example.

Another meaning of 'statistics' is that of a theoretical/*formal science*; it is a *mathematical* one. Closely related to probability theory, this line of mathematics addresses *random variates* (numerical). Mathematical statistics addresses distribution models for random variates per se, for one; and for another, it addresses (hypothetical) 'samples' – sets of independent realizations of particular random variates – specifically numbers derived from these (sample mean, e.g.), as to their distributions in (hypothetical) sets of independent samples – infinite in number, with sample size remaining the same.

Statistics in this mathematical meaning of the term, in select aspects of it, is to epidemiological, and meta-epidemiological clinical, research as mathematics more broadly – including mathematical statistics – is to physics: it is absolutely essential, indispensable. The epidemiological, or meta-epidemiological clinical, researcher should not presume to be able to delegate the requisite statistics to a 'biostatistician' any more than a physicist presumes to be able to delegate the relevant mathematics to a 'physicomathematician.' Occasional need for statistical consultation is another matter.

It is to be understood, however, that *the formal science of statistics is not the theory of statistical science of the empirical sort*, of epidemiological research, for example. As is implied by the organization of this book, the theory of this particular empirical line of statistical research is predicated on select (terms and) concepts of medicine, empirical science in general, and statistics as a theoretical science. Theoretical statistics thus is one of the necessary preliminaries for the development, presentation, and study of the terms and concepts specific to epidemiological, and meta-epidemiological clinical, research. The general concepts specific to those types of empirical research are, in turn, necessary preliminaries for the rest of the theory,

O. S. Miettinen, *Epidemiological Research: Terms and Concepts*,
DOI 10.1007/978-94-007-1171-6_3, © Springer Science+Business Media B.V. 2011

the principles of the research. (The meaning of 'general' here is: without specificity to particular areas of subject-matter.)

While it is clear that the heavily statistical theory of sample surveys is extrinsic to statistics per se (and to statistico-empirical science also), in particular instances the distinction between statistics per se and statistical science can be somewhat challenging. The Mantel-Haenszel statistics, and the test-based 'confidence interval' also, were developed not in the framework of statistics per se but for the needs in epidemiological research; yet they can be seen to be plain statistics. On the other hand, the Kaplan-Meier-Greenwood statistics for 'survival analysis' have an explicit reference to clinical research. The General Linear Model and its 'generalized' extension (incl. the logistic model) developed as topics within statistics per se; but Cox regression was developed specifically for – and it inherently involves concepts of – empirico-statistical science (clinical trials in it).

Whatever may be intrinsic to statistics, Bayesian statistics included, *theory of inference (inductive) in empirico-statistical science is extrinsic to theoretical statistics.*

I – 3. 2. Mini-dictionary

Where an asterisk (*) is here attached to a term, it indicates the term's inclusion in the I.E.A. dictionary of epidemiology [4].

Alternative hypothesis – See 'Hypothesis' (Note 2).

Analysis – Misnomer for synthesis (of sample realizations of a random variate). (Cf. 'Analysis and synthesis' in sect. I – 2. 2.)

Analysis of covariance – See 'General linear model' (Notes 3 and 4).
    Note: 'Analysed' is not covariance but mean.

Analysis of variance* – See 'General linear model' (Notes 3 and 4).
    Note: 'Analysed' is not variance but mean.

Assumption – In a theoretical development, an adopted premise. (Cf. 'Assumption' in sect. I – 2. 2 and 'Assumptions' in sect. II – 4.)

Asymptotic* – Concerning the model for the distribution of a statistic, the quality that it is exactly correct in the context of an infinite-size sample only; also, concerning a statistic per se, the quality that the model for its distribution is asymptotic.

Bayesian* – See 'Statistics' (Note 1).

Bayes' rule/theorem* – In probability theory, an expression for conditional probability:

$Pr(A|B) = Pr(A \text{ and } B)/Pr(B) = Pr(A)\,Pr(B|A)/[Pr(A)\,Pr(B|A)+Pr(\bar{A})\,(Pr(B|\bar{A})].$

*Bernoulli distribution** – The distribution of a random variate (Y) the possible realizations of which are $Y = 0$ and $Y = 1$. A particular distribution of this type is defined by $P = Pr(Y = 1)$, the mean of the distribution. The probability-distribution model thus is:

$$Pr(Y = y) = P^y\,(1-P)^{1-y} \text{ (for } y = 0, 1).$$

The variance of the distribution is $P(1-P)$. (Cf. 'Binomial distribution.')

*Bias** – Concerning a sample-based counterpart of a parameter (an 'estimate' of it, i.e.) in a model for the distribution of a random variate, the extent to which it typically deviates from the corresponding theoretical value (in hypothetical replications of the sampling, independently, at the same amount, ad infinitum).

Note: Usually addressed in statistics is *mean* bias, even though generally more meaningful is *median* bias. The reason for the focus on mean bias is that it generally is amenable to statistical mathematics, while median bias tends not to be. Example: A ratio of two empirical proportions, p_1/p_0, as a measure of the ratio P_1/P_0 of two Bernoulli parameters has an infinite mean bias but (practically) no median bias. The mean bias is infinite because $p_0 = 0$ – and hence $p_1/p_0 = \infty$ – occurs with non-zero probability.

*Binomial distribution** – The distribution of the sum of (the realizations of) N independent and identical Bernoulli variates.

Note: The possible realizations of a binomial random variate (Y) are the integers in the range from 0 to N; and

$$Pr(Y = y) = \binom{N}{y} P^y (1-P)^{N-y} \text{ (for } 0 \leq y \leq N),$$

where P is the mean of each of the Bernoulli variates, and $\binom{N}{y}$ is N combinatorial y. (See 'Combinatorial.') The mean of the distribution is NP, and its variance is $NP(1-P)$.

Binomial model – See 'Binomial distribution.'

*Biometry** (synonym: biostatistics) – See 'Biostatistics.'

*Biostatistics** (synonym: biometry) – 'Applied' statistics relevant to biological research (incl. biomedical research).

Note: There is no single, select body of statistics (mathematical) equally relevant to all biological sciences. Example: The statistics relevant to quintessentially 'applied' epidemiological and related clinical research differs profoundly from statistics relevant to research in, e.g., genetics.

Central limit theorem – The distribution of the sum of the realizations in a sample from whatever distribution (a binomial sample from a Bernoulli distribution, say) is asymptotically Gaussian – with mean NM and variance NV, where N is the size of the sample (N → ∞) and M and V are, respectively, the mean and the variance of the sampled distribution. For the sample mean, correspondingly, the asymptotic distribution is Gaussian with mean M and variance V/N.

Note: Even with a Bernoulli distribution, quite closely Gaussian distribution obtains for the sum and the mean (especially if $P \cong 0.5$) with quite modest N already.

*Chi-squared distribution** – The distribution of the square of a standard-Gaussian (random) variate or statistic, or of the sum of two or more independent standard-Gaussian variates/statistics. The number of standard-Gaussian variates/statistics involved is the number of *degrees of freedom* of a chi-squared, χ^2, distribution.

Note: Concerning random variates, the chi-squared distribution with 1 d.f. is a useless supplement to the standard-Gaussian model; and the chi-squared distribution with more than 1 d.f. is a useless supplement to the Gaussian model for the sum of the unsquared variates. Multi-d.f. χ^2 distributions are useful models for certain statistics only, for their sampling distributions. Example: the statistic in the F test.

Chi-squared model – See 'Chi-squared distribution.'

*Chi-squared test** – A statistical test (of a null hypothesis) in which the test statistic is taken to have (approximately) a chi-squared (χ^2) distribution (with a given number of degrees of freedom, as its sampling distribution), conditionally on the tested value of the parameter at issue.

Note: With d.f. = 1, use of the statistic's square root (with the appropriate sign) amounts to the corresponding Gaussian test.

*Collinearity** – Concerning two or more variates (regressors, notably), their mutual correlatedness, very high correlatedness in particular.

Combinatorial (synonym: binomial coefficient) – The number of different samples/sets of a given size (n) that can be drawn from a larger set of a given size (N).

Note 1: The common notations for this number, for 'N combinatorial n,' are $\binom{N}{n}$, C(N, n) and $^{N}C_{n}$. The value of this combinatorial is N! / n! (N − n)!, where, say, N! is the 'N factorial,' meaning

$$N! = N(N - 1)(N - 2)\ldots \times 2 \times 1.$$

Of note: 0! = 1 (so that N combinatorial N equals 1 – implying that only one distinct sample of size N can be drawn from a set of size N).

Note 2: Combinatorials are eminent in binomial, hypergeometric, and Poisson models.

*Confidence interval** – In frequentist statistics, an interval derived (as a statistic from a random sample) in such a way that with a defined long-term frequency such an interval covers the parameter's (unknown) value.

Note: The term is a misnomer, as 'confidence' is not a frequentist term. The proper term would be *'frequency interval.'*

*Continuous variate** – A variate whose possible realizations in the range of these include all (rather than merely integer) numbers in this range. (Cf. 'Discrete variate.')

*Correlation coefficient** – Concerning the joint distribution of two variates, their covariance divided by the square root of the product of their respective variances (i.e., by the product of their standard deviations).

Covariance – Concerning the joint distribution of two variates, the mean of the product of their respective deviations from their means.

*Covariate** – Concerning a given variate, an associated other variate considered jointly with it; in regression models, all of the independent variates (Xs) are termed covariates (of the dependent variate, Y).

*Dependent variate** – In a regression model, the regressed variate (Y), the mean of which is addressed by the model. (Cf. 'General linear model.')

Descriptive statistic – A statistic derived without any statistical model.

Deviance statistic – In (multiple) regression analysis with ML fitting, and with log-likelihoods L_1 and L_0 with the inclusion and exclusion, respectively, of one or more terms, the difference, $L_1 - L_0$, multiplied by 2. (See 'Deviance test.')

Deviance test – Test of statistical significance of improved fit resulting from adding one or more terms into a regression model. The realization of the deviance statistic is referred to chi-square distribution with degrees of freedom equal to the difference in the number of parameters between the two models. (See 'Deviance statistic.')

*Discrete variate** – A variate whose possible realizations include only the integer numbers in the range of these (incl. the limit numbers).

*Distribution** – Concerning a random variate or a statistic, its possible realizations together with the respective probabilities of, or probability densities at, these; also: concerning a random or a non-random variate, its realizations (in a sample) together with the frequencies of these (in the sample).

Note 1: Those two distributions are termed *sampling* and *sample* distribution, respectively.

Note 2: It would be a nice routine to use for random variates a symbol different from that for non-random ones, notably (as here) Y and X, respectively, and a different symbol yet for a statistic, Z perhaps. At present, X is a common symbol for any random variate, and Z commonly denotes, specifically, a Gaussian test statistic, while Y is commonly used for the dependent variate in a regression model. (Cf. 'General linear model.')

Distribution function* – Concerning a random variate (Y), $\Pr(Y \leq y)$ for all values of y in the range for realizations of the variate.

Note: This customary definition is less than felicitous. In the context of a continuous variate, $\Pr(Y = y) = 0$ for each $Y = y$, and therefore a preferable definition involves, simply, $\Pr(Y < y)$. And in the context of a discrete variate, the cumulative probability has a 'jump' at each one of the realizations $Y = y$, so that at $Y = y$ it actually has a range from $\Pr(Y < y)$ to $\Pr(Y \leq y)$.

Effect* – A parameter's deviation from its null value. (Cf. 'Main effect' and 'Interaction.')

Note: The ubiquitous use of this term – and related ones such as 'main effect' and 'interaction' – in statistics, without any implication of causality, is a strong indication of statistics – like mathematics in general – having developed externally to empirical sciences (cf. sect. I – 3. 1).

Efficient – Concerning a type of statistic (a 'point estimator,' notably), the quality of abstracting the entirety of the information in the data.

Note: The likelihood function is the epitome of an efficient statistic.

Error* – Concerning a realization of a random variate, its deviation from its mean as specified, notably, by the regression model at issue.

Note: The term is a misnomer, falsely implying that the realizations of a random variate are, quite generally, erroneous (the mean being a possible exception to this).

Estimate* – Concerning the value/magnitude (unknown) of a parameter (of the distribution of a random variate), a statistic derived as a measure of this (in frequentist statistics); also: a belief (subjective) about this value, updated by a suitable statistic (the likelihood function, in Bayesian statistics).

Note 1: An estimate is either a *point* estimate – a single possible value of the parameter – or an *interval* estimate – a range of the parameter's possible values. A point estimate is, in a particular, expressly defined sense (maximum-likelihood, say), the 'best bet' of what the parameter's value actually is. A frequentist point estimate is not termed a confidence point; but incongruously with this, a frequentist interval estimate is alternatively (and commonly yet unjustly) termed confidence interval. (Cf. Note under 'Confidence interval.')

Note 2: As the concepts estimation and estimate generally are judgmental in nature (cf. 'Estimation'/'Assessment' in sect. I – 1. 2), 'estimation' and 'estimate' in frequentist terms are *misnomers*, whether in reference to a point or an interval. (In statistical science, a parameter's empirical value is the study result in respect to that parameter, and the width of its associated 'confidence interval' is a measure of its imprecision.)

Note 3: Ideally, all estimates would be viewed as intervals, so that point estimate would be a 0% two-sided interval estimate (of zero width). As it is, point and interval 'estimates' are addressed, in frequentist statistics, not only separately but in ways that are disjoint.

Note 4: A frequentist $100(1 - \alpha)\%$ 'estimate' – interval 'estimate' – is one derived in such a way that $100(\alpha/2)\%$ of the time – in this long-run proportion of instances – the lower limit is too high and, also, another $100(\alpha/2)\%$ of the time the upper limit is too low; that is, this interval covers, in this particular meaning, the parameter's actual value in $100(1 - \alpha)\%$ of the samplings. (Cf. 'Confidence interval.') A 0% 'estimate' in this meaning is median unbiased by definition.

Note 5: A Bayesian $100(1 - \alpha)\%$ interval estimate is one that is taken by someone to contain the parameter's value with probability (subjective) $100(1 - \alpha)\%$, with $100\alpha/2$ probability for each of the two ranges outside this interval estimate. (Cf. Note 4 above.)

Note 6: A frequentist $100(1 - \alpha)\%$ interval 'estimate' is a Bayesian $100(1 - \alpha)\%$ confidence/probability – 'credible' – interval in the context of an ignorance prior only.

Note 7: It would be good of frequentists to replace the word 'estimate' by 'result' in those 'point estimate' and 'interval estimate' terms of theirs.

*Estimator** – Frequentist term for a particular type of function of the data, the realization of which is the corresponding 'estimate' (in the frequentist meaning of 'estimate'; see Notes under 'Estimate').

*Exact P-value** – A P-value derived under the actual model for a discrete distribution (rather than an asymptotic approximation to this), a model such as a binomial, Poisson, or hypergeometric one. (See 'Hypergeometric test,' incl. Fisher's exact test under it, and also 'Mid-P.')

Note 1: The term is a misnomer, as the resulting P-value, especially as it ordinarily is derived (e.g., from the Fisher 'exact' test), does not have the null distribution of uniform 0-to-1 (so that $\Pr[P < \alpha = \alpha])$; and besides, as P-value from the test's 'inexact' (asymptotic) counterpart is asymptotically exact – and as that from the t test, for example, is also is exact whenever its model is satisfied.

Note 2: An 'exact' P-value generally is inexact also in the meaning that the sum of the upper-tail and lower-tail P-values exceeds unity (by the amount of the probability of the observed realization). The use of the mid-P solves this problem.

*Exact test** – A statistical test (of a null hypothesis) involving the derivation of the 'exact' P-value – generally inexact though this actually is (cf. 'Exact P-Value.')

Expectation (synonyms: expected value, mean) – Concerning a random variate or a statistic, the mean of its distribution.

Note: The term is a gross misnomer, as one cannot – realistically, and in general – expect the realization from a distribution to turn out to be the mean of this distribution. For example, in the case of a Bernoulli (0, 1) variate, one can expect its realization to be the mean, P, only in the 'degenerate' cases of $P = 0$ and $P = 1$.

F-distribution* – Concerning two independent statistics Z_1 and Z_2, having chi-squared distributions with d_1 and d_2 degrees of freedom, respectively, the distribution of (Snedecor's) $F = (Z_1/d_1) / (Z_2/d_2)$ – this distribution being the F distribution with d_1 and d_2 degrees of freedom, $F(d_1, d_2)$.

Note: Sample variance, with $N - 1$ d.f., divided by the variance, V, of the sampled Gaussian distribution, has χ^2 distribution with $N - 1$ d.f. Hence the use of an F-test to address tenability of the homscedasticity premise in a model and/or the magnitude of the variance ratio.

Fisher's exact test* – See 'Hypergeometric test' (Note 3).

Frequentism/frequentist – See 'Statistics' (Note 1).

F-test* (synonym: variance-ratio test) – Statistical test of homoscedasticity (by the use of an F-distributed statistic). (See 'F-distribution.')

Function* – A mathematical expression for the way in which one quantity depends on another or, jointly, on a set of others. (Example: regression model.)

Gaussian distribution* (synonym: normal distribution) – The distribution in which the possible realizations are all real numbers (from $-\infty$ to $+\infty$), and for which the probability-density at any given $Y = y$ is

$$f(y) = (1/2\pi V)^{1/2} \exp[-(y - M)^2/2V] \text{ (for } -\infty \le y \le +\infty),$$

where M and V are, respectively, the mean and the variance of the distribution. Analogously for any given $Z = z$ (see Note 2 under 'Distribution').

Note 1: $\Pr(Y = y) = 0$ for each y, while $\Pr(y_1 < Y < y_2)$ for any $y_1 < y_2$ is the integral of $f(y)$ from y_1 to y_2.

Note 2: The Gaussian distribution with $M = 0$ and $V = 1$ is termed the *standard-Gaussian* distribution. Its 95th centile is 1.96, used for 95% 'confidence intervals.'

Note 3: A sample-based counterpart of a parameter is generally taken to have, asymptotically, a Gaussian distribution (sampling-distribution), per the Central Limit Theorem.

Gaussian model – See 'Gaussian distribution.'

Gaussian test – Statistical test (of a null hypothesis) in which the test statistic is taken to have (approximately) the standard-Gaussian distribution (on the null hypothesis).

Note: This term – patterned after the well-established 't test' and 'χ^2 test' – is a here-adduced neologism.

General linear model (GLM) – Formulation of the mean/'expectation' of (the distribution of) a random variate (Y) as a linear compound of a set $\{B_i\}$ of parameters: as $B_0 + \sum_i B_i X_i$.

Note 1: Y is the dependent variate, while the Xs are independent variates. (Y is random, the Xs possibly non-random).

Note 2: A *linear compound* of a set of quantities is, by definition (in mathematics), of the form $L = \sum_i C_i Q_i$, where the $\{Q_i\}$ are the quantities at issue and the $\{C_i\}$ are their respective coefficients in the linear compound, L. In the GLM here, the Xs – the independent variates (incl. $X_0 \equiv 1$) – are the coefficients of the quantities $\{B_i\}$. The GLM is 'linear in the parameters,' in this meaning of 'linear.'

Note 3: The GLM was introduced (in the 1950s) as a unification of 'analysis of *variance*,' 'analysis of *covariance*,' and '*regression* analysis.' This is the sense in which the GLM is general. The distinctions were seen to be (merely) matters of the nature of the Xs, namely: all indicator variates, a combination of indicator and quantitative variates, and all quantitative variates, respectively.

Note 4: The GLM is now termed a *regression* model regardless of the nature of the Xs (i.e., regardless of whether they are all indicator variates, all quantitative variates, or a mixture of these).

Note 5: The GLM, while already general in the meaning of Note 3 above, got to be generalized (in the 1970s) into the *Generalized* linear model. By this further generalization, the dependent parameter need not be the mean of Y as such; it can be a transform (metameter) of this (as, e.g., in the models for logistic regression).

Generalized linear model – See 'General linear model' (Note 5).

GLM – General linear model, or generalized linear model.

*Homoscedasticity** – Constancy of variance (theoretical) across a set of categories.

*Hypergeometric distribution** – The distribution of a binomial random variate conditionally on the sum of this binomial and another, independent binomial with the same value for the Bernoulli parameter. This is to say: if $Y_1 \sim B(N_1, P)$ and, independently, $Y_0 \sim B(N_0, P)$, then $(Y_1 | Y_1 + Y_0 = M_1) \sim H(N_1, N_0, M_1)$. (See 'Non-central hypergeometric distribution.')

Note 1: The range of the possible values of Y_1 is max $(0, M_1 - N_0) \leq Y_1 \leq$ min (M_1, N_1). The probability of $Y_1 = y_1$, within this range, is

$$Pr(Y_1 = y_1) = C(N_1, y_1)\, C(N_0, M_1 - y_1)/C(N_1 + N_0, M_1),$$

where, for example, $C(N_1, y_1)$ is 'N_1 combinatorial y_1,' meaning $N!/y_1!(N_1 - y_1)!$

Note 2: The mean and variance of Y_1 are, respectively, $M_1 N_1/(N_1 + N_0)$ and $M_1 M_0 N_1 N_0/N^2(N - 1)$, where $N = M_1 + M_0 = N_1 + N_0$.

Hypergeometric model – See 'Hypergeometric distribution.'

Hypergeometric test – Statistical test of identity of two probabilities (Bernoulli parameters) under the hypergeometric model.

Note 1: Given the binomial proportions y_1/N_1 and y_0/N_0, with $y_1 + y_0 = M_1$, $N_1 + N_0 = N$, and $M_0 = N - M_1$, the *asymptotic* test statistic (hypergeometric) is

$(y_1 - M_1 N_1 / N) / [M_1 M_0 N_1 N_0 / N^2 (N - 1)]^{1/2}.$

Its realization is referred to a table of the standard-Gaussian distribution (to obtain the null P-value). Alternatively, the square of this statistic is referred to a table of the chi-square distribution with 1 d.f. (Cf. 'Hypergeometric distribution,' Note 2, and see 't test,' Note 5.)

Note 2: When the asymptotic model is not justifiable, the corresponding *'exact'* test needs to be deployed (under the hypergeometric model). The null mid-P-value is

$$(^1/_2) \Pr(Y_1 = y_1) + \Pr(Y_1 > y_1),$$

if the alternative hypothesis is $P_1 > P_0$; otherwise the P-value is the complement of this. The probabilities of the realizations of Y_1 are the hypergeometric ones. (See 'Hypergeometric distribution.')

Note 3: When using $\Pr(Y_1 = y_1)$ in lieu of half of this, the calculation of the null P-value is known as *Fisher's exact* test. (Cf. 'Exact P-value.')

Note 4: 'Hypergeometric test' is a here-adduced neologism (cf. Note under 'Gaussian test').

*Hypothesis** – Concerning a parameter in a model for the distribution of a variate or a statistic, a value, or a range of values, of it considered in inference about the parameter's value/magnitude (unknown).

Note 1: At issue commonly is a parameter that has to do with the mean of a dependent variate (Y) in respect to its possible dependence on one of the independent variates (Xs). (Cf. 'Model,' Note 2.)

Note 2: In the case addressed by Note 1 above, of particular interest most commonly is the simple possibility that the dependence is non-existent, that the value/magnitude of the parameter is zero. This possibility is termed the *null* hypothesis, and a given one of the other possibilities, or all of these in the aggregate, is said to constitute the *alternative* hypothesis.

Note 3: The null hypothesis may address a set of parameters jointly. If the mean of the dependent variate is hypothesized to be dependent on something specified on a nominal scale, and this potential dependence is modeled by means of indicator Xs in a regression model (one fewer than the number of categories), of interest may be the *omnibus null hypothesis* that all of the parameters (Bs) associated with these Xs are zero – that the hypothesized nominal-scale determinant of the mean of Y actually affords no meaningful distinctions according to the *'multiple'* (more than one) contrasts that are possible to make.

Note 4: The statistical concept of hypothesis – inclusive of null 'hypothesis' – is at variance with that in science (cf. sect. I – 2. 2).

Hypothesis testing – Given a sample from the distribution of a random variate, derivation from it of a statistic and translation of this into inference about the correctness/incorrectness of the (null) hypothesis. (See 'Significance testing.')

Note 1: The frequentist statistic in hypothesis testing is the null P-value, based on the realization of a test statistic, while the Bayesian statistic is the likelihood function (of the parameter at issue).

Note 2: The null P-value together with the parameter's sample value imply the likelihood function (for Bayesian inference).

*Independent variate** – In a regression model, any particular one of the regressor variates (Xs). (Cf. 'General linear model.')

*Inference** – Concerning a parameter in a statistical model, the deployment of the sample realization of an inferential statistic to arrive at an updated belief about the magnitude of the parameter at issue.

Note 1: Given that at issue in genuine inference is belief, its inputs cannot be statistics alone; inference requires the framework that includes *subjective* probability (cf. 'Estimate,' Note 2). Thus, only Bayesian statistics actually addresses the theory of statistical inference (a point not recognized/admitted by frequentists).

Note 2: Given that frequentist 'inferential' statistics imply the Bayesian one (see 'Statistics,' Note 2), the frequentist statistics can be used for inference (in the proper, Bayesian meaning of this).

Note 3: In respect to hypothesis-testing, frequentist 'inference' has been a matter of statistic-driven (P-value-based) *conclusion* about acceptance/rejection of the (null) hypothesis; but, incongruously, there has not been the counterpart of this in 'estimation' – acceptance/rejection of particular range(s) of non-null values of the parameter at issue. (Cf. 'Confidence interval.')

Inferential statistic – A statistic derived under a statistical model.

*Information** – Concerning a sample, the extent to which a 'point estimate' of a parameter from it generally reflects the true, theoretical value of the parameter – specifically in the sense of the inverse of the 'mean square error' in the distribution of the 'point estimate' of the parameter.

*Interaction** – The needed involvement, in the linear compound of a regression model, a term in which ($B_i \neq 0$ and) the X_i is a product of two other Xs in the compound.

Note: The term is a misnomer for the concept. For, at issue is merely the way in which the mean of the dependent variate (Y) depends on the Xs, considered jointly, and not any interaction between the Xs (one influencing the other, and conversely, as in: Love makes time pass, time makes love pass.) (Cf. 'Effect' and 'Main effect.')

Intercept – In a GLM, the value (B_0) of the linear compound when $X_i = 0$ for all $i \neq 0$. (Cf. 'Slope.')

*Interval estimate** – See 'Estimate' (Notes 1-6).

Level of test – An a-priori 'critical' value (α) in frequentist hypothesis/significance testing, such that $P < α$ is deemed 'significant' (at level α) and $P > α$ 'non-significant' in the sense of calling, respectively, for 'rejection' and 'acceptance' of the null 'hypothesis.'

Note 1: By analogy, then, a $100 (1 - α)\%$ 'interval estimate' or 'confidence interval' should be taken to contain the values of the parameter that are 'accepted' at 'level α,' with those outside this interval 'rejected' at that 'level.'

Note 2: Frequentist theory of 'inference' leaves unclear who it is whose decision (*sic*) is at issue.

*Likelihood function** – Concerning the realization of the 'sufficient' statistic in the context of the (statistical) model for the distribution of this, the probability of, or probability-density at, the realization of the statistic as a function of the magnitude of a parameter in the model.

Linear – See 'General linear model' (Note 2).

*Logistic model** – Generalized linear model for the mean (*M*) of a Bernoulli variate (Y), one in which the linear formulation is given to the logit transform of the mean of Y; that is, to $\log[M/(1 - M)]$. (See 'Model.')

Note: Implied by this linear formulation for the logit of *M* is that *M* itself is a non-linear function of the parameters (the *B*s):

$$M = 1/\{1 + \exp\left[- \left(B_0 + \Sigma_i B_i X_i\right)\right]\}.$$

Logistic regression – Regression 'analysis' in the framework of a logistic model.

*Logit** – Logarithm (natural) of odds.

Main effect – In a GLM, concerning a particular one (X_i) of the independent variates which is not a product of two (or more) of the others, the (magnitude of the) parameter (B_i) associated with it.

Note: In statistical jargon, all regression parameters represent 'effects,' without any inherent meaning of causality. (Cf. 'Effect' and 'Interaction.')

*Maximum likelihood** – The quality of a point 'estimate' (in frequentist statistics) of corresponding to the maximum of the likelihood function.

Mean bias (synonym: bias) – Concerning a point 'estimator,' the quality of the mean of its (sampling) distribution not coinciding with the value of the parameter being 'estimated'; also: the magnitude of this discrepancy.

Mean square error – Concerning the realizations of a point 'estimator,' in hypothetical replications of the sampling, independently, at the same size, an infinite number of times, the mean of the realizations' squared deviations from the parameter's actual value. (It thus is the sum of sampling variance and the square of the mean bias.)

Median bias – Concerning a point 'estimator,' the quality of the median of its (sampling) distribution not coinciding with the value of the parameter being 'estimated'; also: the magnitude of this discrepancy.

Mid-P – 'Exact' P-value modified by including only half of the probability of the observed realization. (See 'Exact P-value.')

Note 1: When using, as remains commonplace, the full probability of the observed realization for the statistic at issue, the sum of the 'upper-tail' and 'lower-tail' P-values exceeds one, which should not happen. Use of the mid-P removes this problem (cf. Note 2 under 'Exact P-value'). Mid-P also has more closely the intended property that $Pr(P < \alpha|H_0) = \alpha$, H_0 denoting the null 'hypothesis.'

Note 2: If the idea is that $P = 0.50$ should correspond to the ML point 'estimate,' then in the context of a Poisson model the 'upper-tail' P-value should involve the multiplier 2/3 for the observed realization, while for the 'lower-tail' P-value the corresponding multiplier is 1/3. (These multipliers are exactly correct only asymptotically.)

ML – Maximum likelihood.

*Model** – Concerning a distribution (of a random variate or a statistic), a mathematical expression defining the probabilities of, or probability-densities at, each of the possible realizations, the way these depend on the parameter(s) in the model. (Example: a logistic extension of the Bernoulli model.)

Note 1: A model in this meaning actually is an infinite number of models, each of these corresponding to some particular value(s) of the parameter(s).

Note 2: The essence of a *regression* model is the way in which the mean of the dependent variate (Y) is formulated as a joint function of the independent variates (Xs) being considered.

Note 3: The logistic model is a generalized Bernoulli model in the sense that it defines (the form of) the way the sole parameter (mean) of this is thought to be a function of the set of Xs in the model (the way the single parameter of the Bernoulli distribution depends on the Xs).

*Multicollinearity** – In multiple-regression 'analysis,' one regressor's correlatedness with a linear compound of (some of) the others, very high correlatedness in particular.

*Multiple-comparison problem** – In 'analysis of variance,' the result of (i.e., the null P-value from) the proper test statistic concerning the omnibus null 'hypothesis' is not reproduced by tests specific to particular other comparisons between/among the categories (nominal) involved.

*Multiple regression** – Regression 'analysis' with two or more regressors (independent variates) in the model.

*Multivariate regression** – Regression 'analysis' with two or more regressands (dependent variates) in the model.

Non-central hypergeometric distribution – Generalization of the hypergeometric distribution to the (non-null) case of $P_1 \neq P_0$. (Cf. 'Hypergeometric distribution.')

Note 1: The range of the distribution is, of course, the same as that of the hypergeometric distribution, and

$$Pr(Y_1 = y_1) = \frac{C(N_1, y_1) \, C(N_0, M_1 - y_1)(OR)y_1}{\sum_i (N_1, i)C \, (N_0, M_1 - i)(OR)^i},$$

where $OR = [P/(1 - P_1)]/[P_0/(1 - P_0)]$, the non-centrality parameter (odds ratio), and the summation is over the range of Y_1 (see 'Hypergeometric distribution').

Note 2: The mean, M, of the distribution and the OR have, asymptotically, this relation:

$$OR = M(M_0 - N_1 + M)/(M_1 - M) \, (N_1 - M),$$

and the asymptotic variance of its logarithm is, to a first-order Taylor series approximation,

$$V = M^{-1} + (M_1 - M)^{-1} + (N_1 - M)^{-1} + (M_0 - N_1 + M)^{-1}.$$

*Normal distribution** (synonym: Gaussian distribution) – See 'Gaussian distribution.'

Nuisance parameter – An extraneous parameter that needs to be 'estimated' in 'estimation' of the parameter of interest. (Example: mean in the 'estimation' of variance.)

*Null hypothesis** – See 'Hypothesis' (Notes 2 and 3).

Null P-value – See 'P-value' (Notes 2-4).

*Odds** – Probability (P) divided by its complement $(1 - P)$; that is, $P/(1 - P)$.

Omnibus null hypothesis – In 'analysis of variance,' the null 'hypothesis' that all of the means (of Y) are identical. (Cf. 'Hypothesis,' Note 3).

*Parameter** – A constant (of unknown magnitude) in a (statistical) model. (Cf. 'Parameter' in sect. I – 1. 2.)

Point estimate – See 'Estimate' (Notes 1, 3 and 7).

*Poisson distribution** – The limit of the binomial distribution as $N \to \infty$ and $P \to 0$ with NP remaining finite.

Note: The possible realizations of a Poisson variate (Y) are all non-negative integers (from 0 to ∞); and

$$\Pr(Y = y) = [\exp(-M)]M^y/y! \ (0 \le y \le \infty),$$

where M is the mean (and variance) of the distribution (equal to NP) and y! is the y factorial. (See 'Combinatorial,' Note 1.)

*Posterior** (synonym: posterior distribution) – The result of a prior distribution's updating in the face of a set of data (in Bayesian inference). (See 'Prior.')

*Power** – Concerning a test of statistical significance in a given application (prospective, with its given sample size), $\Pr(P < \alpha|\Delta)$, where P is the null P-value, α is the level of significance chosen for the test (a value in the 0-to-1 range, commonly $\alpha = 0.05$), and Δ is a possible degree to which the parameter at issue might deviate from its null value (as one possible value of the deviation). (See 'Sample size determination.')

*Prior** (synonym: prior distribution) – In Bayesian statistics, the distribution of someone's probability (subjective) for various ranges of the value/magnitude of the parameter at issue prior to the update of this in the face of an available set of data (the likelihood function derived from these).
  Note: A generally suitable way to specify a prior is the cumulative probability of this as a function of the parameter at issue. In this, the null value of the parameter is commonly associated with a 'jump' in the (cumulative) probability.

*Probability** – See 'Statistics.'

*Probability density** – Concerning a possible value (y) in the distribution of a continuous random variate (Y), the limit of $\Pr(y < Y < y + \Delta)/\Delta$ as $\Delta \to 0$. It is the derivative of the (cumulative) distribution function of Y at $Y = y$.

*Probability sample** – Sample resulting from probability sampling.

*Probability sampling** – Sampling in such a way that each member of the sampled set of units has a known and independent probability of getting to be selected into the sample.

*P-value** – A statistic so derived (from a sample) that its (sampling) distribution conditional on the parameter value being tested is uniform in the 0-to-1 range, so that $\Pr(P < \alpha) = \alpha$ for any α in this range; and so derived that, in addition, the distribution on the 'alternative' hypothesis is shifted to the left in this same range, so that $\Pr(P < \alpha) > \alpha$.
  Note 1: That pair of distributions for the P-value statistic is achieved by deriving this statistic as either the cumulative probability at the test statistic's realization or as the complement of this, conditionally on the value of the parameter being tested. The choice between these two options – the 'lower-tail' and 'upper-tail' P-value – is made so as to achieve the distribution's shift to the left rather than to the right on the alternative hypothesis.

Note 2: Meant by *the* P-value generally is the *null P-value*, associated with testing of the null 'hypothesis.'

Note 3: It remains commonplace to define the P-value not by its distributional properties (as above and elsewhere [12]) but by the way it is derived – as a probability (Note 1 above). An unfortunate consequence of this is the common misconception that the null P-value is the probability that the null 'hypothesis' is true (cf. Preface).

Note 4: It is not inherent in the concept of a P-value that, in the context of a test statistic with a discrete distribution, the full probability of the statistic's realization enters into the cumulative probability (cf. Note 1 above). Always better than this is use of only half of this probability (in the 'mid-P'); but even this can be improved upon, so as to assure 0.50 to be the value of the P-value function at what is taken to be the best – the 'maximum likelihood' – point 'estimate' of – the point result on – the parameter at issue. (Cf. 'Mid-P.')

P-value function – P-value as a function of all possible values of the parameter (as conceivable values to be tested).

Note: This function [12] implies all of the usual frequentist statistics: the null P-value, the point 'estimate' (corresponding to $P = 0.50$), and the $100(1 - \alpha)\%$ confidence' limits (corresponding to $P = \alpha/2$ and $P = 1 - \alpha/2$, respectively).

*Random sample** (synonym: probability sample) – See 'Probability sample.'

*Random variable**/variate– See 'Variate.'

Realization – Concerning a random variate or a statistic, its value in a particular instance.

*Regressand** – In a regression model, the dependent variate (Y), or the mean of this, or a transform of the mean.

Regression coefficient – In a regression model, the parameter (B_i) associated with a given one of the independent variates (X_i, incl. the B_0 coefficient of $X_0 \equiv 1$).

*Regressor** – In a regression model, a given one of the independent variates (Xs).

*Sample** – A set of realizations of a random variate.

Sample distribution – See 'Distribution' (Note 1).

*Sample size determination** – Calculation of the sample size (N) which, in the context of a given level of the test of statistical significance, would imply a given level $(1 - \beta)$ of power in the context of a given deviation (Δ) from the null state.

*Sampling** – The acquisition of a sample (of realizations of a random variate).

Sampling distribution – See 'Distribution' (Note 1).

Scalar – See 'Variate' (Note 2).

SD – Standard deviation.

SE – Standard error.

*Significance** – See 'Statistical significance.'

Simple regression – Regression 'analysis' with only one independent variate in the model.

Slope – In a GLM, concerning a particular one (X_i) of the independent variates (other than $X_0 \equiv 1$), the parameter (B_i) associated with it. (Cf. 'Intercept.')

*Standard deviation** – The square root (positive) of variance.
   Note: An SD is meaningful (as a measure of scatter) only in the context of a (near-) Gaussian distribution (as SD is involved only in Gaussian models).

*Standard error** – An 'estimate' (frequentist point 'estimate') of the SD of the sampling distribution of a sample value (point 'estimate') of a parameter.
   Note 1: An SE, like an SD, is meaningful (for interpretation) only in the context of a (near-) Gaussian distribution. (See 'Wald statistic.')
   Note 2: An SE should involve the unbiased rather than than ML 'estimate' of variance (cf. Notes 2-5 under 't test.')

Standard-Gaussian distribution – See 'Gaussian distribution' (Note 2).

Statistic – A number derived from a sample. See 'Descriptive statistic' and 'Inferential statistic.'

*Statistical significance** – In frequentist hypothesis-testing, the extent to which the sample is consistent with the null 'hypothesis' – as measured by the null P-value.

*Statistics** – The theoretical science (branch of mathematics) that addresses random variates – the distributions of these under particular models and inference about the parameters of the models of these distributions (on the basis of 'statistics' derived from samples from these distributions); also: the art of the acquisition and presentation of aggregate data on the populations of various jurisdictional units (countries, say). (Cf. sect. I – 3. 1.)
   Note 1: The theory of statistical inference (about parameters of distributions of random variates) is (very) different between *frequentist* and *Bayesian** statistics. At the root of this duality is a profound difference in the conception of *probability.** To a frequentist, probability has to do, solely, with a possible future occurrence (of an

event or a state); and it is the 'long-term' relative frequency of this outcome's occurrence, the proportion of the instances ('experiments of chance') at issue in general
such that the outcome will occur. To a Bayesian, this relative frequency is but one
of two concepts of probability, the *objective* one. It pertains to models for distributions of random variates and statistics (as with frequentists). Inputs to inference
in Bayesian statistics involve not only sample-derived statistics but also, centrally,
the other, *subjective* type of probability: the degree of belief about the value of a
parameter being in a given range (of its possible values). Statistical inference is,
to a Bayesian, about updating such beliefs (objectively) in the light of the relevant
inferential statistic (assumed to be valid).

Note 2: The frequentist inferential statistics – null P-value, point and interval
'estimates' – are all implicit in P-value as a function of the parameter [12], while the
P-value function's counterpart in Bayesian statistics is the *likelihood (or likelihood-
ratio) function* of the parameter. The latter implies the former, and vice versa.
Thus, the frequentist-Bayesian duality is not materially one of types of statistics
derived from samples, but one of the deployment of statistics in inference – genuine
inference in Bayesian terms only. (Cf. 'Inference.')

*Test** – In statistical hypothesis-testing, the derivation from the sample of a statistic
(inferential) as a measure of the statistical significance of the sample as pointing to
the null 'hypothesis' not being true (in frequentist statistics) or for inference about
the correctness/incorrectness of the hypothesis (in Bayesian statistics).

Test statistic – The statistic used in statistical hypothesis-testing, capturing the
essence of the sample data for the purpose.

*t test** – In the two-sample context, a test of statistical significance of the difference
between the two means under the model: independent Gaussian distributions of the
respective random variates, having identical (but unknown) variances. The (null)
test statistic is

$$t = (\bar{y}_1 - \bar{y}_0) \Big/ \left[\frac{SS_1 + SS_2}{N_1 + N_2 - 2}(1/N_1 + 1/N_0) \right]^{1/2},$$

where $\bar{y}_1$ and $\bar{y}_0$ are the two sample means, SS_1 and SS_0 are the respective 'sums
of squares' (sums of squared deviations from the respective means, $\bar{y}_1$ and $\bar{y}_0$), and
N_1 and N_0 are the respective sample sizes. The statistic's value is translated into
the corresponding null P-value by reference to a table of the *t distribution* with
$N_1 + N_0 - 2$ degrees of freedom.

Note 1: With increasing number of degrees of freedom, the t distribution
converges – quite quickly – to the standard-Gaussian distribution.

Note 2: With increasing number of degrees of freedom the distribution of the t
statistic converges to the standard-Gaussian distribution even if the distributions of
the two variates (Y_1 and Y_0) are not Gaussian. If the two variates have *Bernoulli*
distributions, the 't statistic' is

$$(\bar{y}_1 - \bar{y}_0)\Big/\left[\frac{N_1\bar{y}_1(1 - \bar{y}_1) + N_0\bar{y}_0(1 - \bar{y}_0)}{N_1 + N_0 - 2}(1/N_1 + 1/N_0)\right]^{1/2}.$$

Its realization can just as well be referred to a table of the standard-Gaussian distribution, as the number of degrees of freedom needs to be appreciable. (At 30 d.f. already, the 97.5 centile of the t distribution is 2.0, as with the standard-Gaussian.) (See Note 4 below.)

Note 3: When homoscedasticity cannot be a feature of the (null) model, the two variances need to be 'estimated' separately. The corresponding statistic now is

$$(\bar{y}_1 - \bar{y}_0)\Big/\left[\frac{SS_1}{(N_1 - 1)N_1} + \frac{SS_0}{(N_0 - 1)N_0}\right]^{1/2}.$$

This is not a t statistic; its realization is referred to a table of the standard-Gaussian distribution.

Note 4: The 't statistic' for testing the significance of the difference between two *Bernoulli* means (Note 2 above) has no raison d'être. A better statistic is

$$(\bar{y}_1 - \bar{y}_0)\Big/\left[\frac{\bar{y}(1 - \bar{y})N}{N - 1}(1/N_1 + 1/N_2)\right]^{1/2},$$

where $\bar{y} = (N_1\bar{y}_1 + N_0\bar{y}_0)/N$ and $N = N_1 + N_0$. Its value is referred to a table of the standard-Gaussian distribution, when N is suitably large.

Note 5: The statistic above (Note 4) is algebraically interchangeable with that of the asymptotic *hypergeometric* test. When N is too small for the asymptotic (Gaussian) model, the exact hypergeometric test is to be used instead.

*Type I error** – In frequentist hypothesis-testing, the rejection of a correct null 'hypothesis.'

*Type II error** – In frequentist hypothesis-testing, the failure to reject an incorrect null 'hypothesis.'

Uniform 0-1 distribution – The distribution of a random variate (Y) the possible realizations of which are all numbers in the 0-to-1 range, the probability density at any given $Y = y, 0 \le y \le 1$, being 1; hence, $Pr(Y \le \alpha) = \alpha$ for any α in the 0-to-1 range. (Cf. P-value.)

*Variable** (synonym: variate) – See 'Variate.'

Note: One might eschew the use of the word 'variable' synonymously with 'variate' on the ground that being variable is an inherent quality of a variate; that 'variable' is an adjective while 'variate' is a noun.

*Variance** – Concerning a random variate or a statistic (frequentist point 'estimate,' most notably), the mean of the squares of its realizations' deviations from the mean of its distribution (sampling distribution, if a statistic).

*Variate** (synonym: variable) – A numerical quantity with a particular set of realizations, possible or actual.

Note 1: A *random* variate is further characterized by a particular model defining the (objective) probability of, or probability-density at, each of the possible realizations. (Cf. 'Distribution.')

Note 2: A random variate need not be unidimensional, a *scalar*; it can have more than one dimension; that is, it can be *vector-valued* (as is the dependent variate in multivariate regression and the independent variate in multiple regression).

Vector – A unidimensional array of quantities (notably variates, realizations of variates, or parameters, e.g., $X_0, X_1, \ldots, X_I$ and $B_0, B_1, \ldots, B_I$).

Wald statistic – A parameter's sample value ('point estimate') divided by its standard error, the realization to be referred to the standard-Gaussian distribution.

Note: This statistic, while in common use – as for regression coefficients, for example – is not a first-principles test-statistic. The SE involves, by its general definition, an 'estimate' of the mean (as a nuisance parameter) and, specifically, the sample value of this. A first-principles test-statistic, by contrast, involves the null counterpart of this (either the 'estimate' of the sampling distribution's SD conditionally on the parameter's null value, or this null SD itself – as in, e.g., the M-H test statistic; sect. II – 4).

PART II
EPIDEMIOLOGICAL RESEARCH PROPER

II – 1. INTRODUCTION

The term *'epidemiological research'* tends to be used, at present, in reference to any research that addresses the rate of occurrence of a phenomenon of 'health' in a human population. There is little or no concern to distinguish between *clinical* research (ultimately on rate-based probabilities, in reference to individuals) and genuinely epidemiological research (on rates per se, concerning populations). No-one seems to ask, for example, whether research in 'pharmaco-epidemiology' actually is epidemiological or, instead, clinical. And the term also is applied to inquiries that are not research at all. At issue may be mere fact-finding (about rates), especially fact-finding that is part of epidemiological practice (of community medicine); and the phenomena being addressed may be ones of healthcare rather than of health.

The I.E.A. dictionary [4] does not define *epidemiology* as community medicine. Instead, the definition it gives is this: "The study of the occurrence and distribution of health-related states or events in specified populations, including the study of the determinants influencing such states [*sic*], and the application of this knowledge to control the health problems." Explications of the terms in this follow, starting with this: "Study includes surveillance, observation, hypothesis-testing, analytic research, and experiments." The closing explication is that "control of health problems" as the aim of epidemiology means "to promote, protect, and restore [*sic*] health." *Epidemiological research* that dictionary defines as: "Occurrence research – i.e., research among people into the frequency of occurrence of phenomena of public health, clinical, social, or biological relevance, with measures of frequency and causal assessments related to the determinants of such phenomena." Much could be said, critically, about these definitions.

Epidemiological research may actually defy definition that is generally agreeable – objective in this meaning. But it definitely is possible to define *quintessentially 'applied'* epidemiological research. This is research to advance the *knowledge-base* of community medicine (cf. Preface) – of epidemiology, that is (cf. sect. I – 1. 2). Advancement of the knowledge-base of community medicine is so important that it generally trumps the rest of the research in this genre, whatever might be someone's definition of the entirety of epidemiological research. As a consequence, epidemiological research is here addressed in terms of that quintessentially 'applied' segment of it, this alone.

O. S. Miettinen, *Epidemiological Research: Terms and Concepts*,
DOI 10.1007/978-94-007-1171-6_4, © Springer Science+Business Media B.V. 2011

Some clarification of this concept and term may be in order. All of truly medical research – so-called 'basic' medical research included – is 'applied' in the meaning that it is conducted in the interest of advancing the practice of medicine [16]. Medical research that is not quintessentially 'applied' holds some promise – quite remote, perhaps – of bringing an innovation – a new tool (a 'biomarker' of some risk, say) or perhaps a newly-established concept (e.g., anti-oxidants as cancer preventives) – for potential deployment, or consideration, in practice. The practitioner need not know about the results of, or even the knowledge derived from, this research, at least not before the new tool or concept arrives. If and when it does arrive, it can enter into the objects of some of the quintessentially 'applied' research, to develop the knowledge-base of its deployment in scientific practice of medicine.

I continue to keep that adjective 'applied' in quotes, to indicate that it is jargon of science that I regard as less than apposite (cf. sect. I – 2. 2). I use the word because it is so deeply and widely ingrained in science, mathematics and statistics included, and because no obviously better alternative has been adduced. It means that the research is not 'pure' – science for the sake of science – but, instead, intended to produce knowledge for some application outside science itself. This suggests that alternatives to consider are 'instrumental' and 'pragmatic' (cf. sect. I – 2. 2).

In 'epidemiological' research, now that it has so dramatically expanded in volume and also in scope, sight has largely been lost of the earlier focus on the advancement of the knowledge-base of community medicine. The component concerns in this community-oriented research could be seen to be the advancements of the knowledge-base for the three types of gnosis – diagnosis, etiognosis, and prognosis – in the epidemiological meanings of these [17].

Community diagnosis, concerning a particular illness, is about its current rate of occurrence in the cared-for population (rate of incidence if at issue is an event, rate of prevalence if at issue is a state; cf. Preface and sect. 1. 2); it is about the illness-specific *morbidity*, current, in the cared-for population (cf. 'Morbidity' in sect. I – 1. 2). Specifically, community diagnosis is *knowing* about the current morbidity from a particular illness in the cared-for community/population, knowing about the *level* of this morbidity (cf. sect. I – 1. 2).

Community etiognosis is about the etiogenesis of the current level of morbidity from a particular illness in the cared-for population. It is *knowing* about the extent to which this morbidity is due to a particular etiogenetic factor (its presence in lieu of its alternative). It is knowing about this etiogenetic fraction/proportion (cf. sect. I – 1. 2).

Community prognosis is about the future course of the morbidity from a particular illness in the cared-for population. It is *knowing* about the future levels of this morbidity in the cared-for population (cf. sect. I – 1. 2).

Research to advance the knowledge-base of community *diagnosis* addresses morbidity (rate of incidence or prevalence) from a particular illness as a function of, mainly, demographic determinants of that level. This concerns non-communicable illnesses only, their endemic levels of morbidity. One alternative to basing community diagnosis on general knowledge about morbidity as a (descriptive) function of its determinants would in principle be a prevalence survey on the cared-for population. This would be a consideration for a relatively chronic illness only. In such a survey (which is not research; cf. sect. II – 2), clinical-diagnostic probability of the presence of the illness would be set for each person-moment in the sample, and the sample prevalence of the illness would be derived as the mean of these probabilities. The incidence counterparts of prevalence surveys are more realistic to consider. They require canvassing the care facilities for the illness at issue, except insofar as cases of the illness are subject to registration. The event at issue here is coming to rule-in diagnosis of the illness at issue, first rule-in diagnosis to be specific.

Research for community *etiognosis* about a particular illness addresses a causal rate-ratio of its occurrence, contrasting the presence of the etiologic/etiogenetic antecedent with that of its alternative; it addresses this parameter conditionally on extraneous determinants of the rate's magnitude, and as a function of its (demographic) modifiers. In practice, such an RR for a particular stratum (demographic) needs to be coupled with particularistic information about the frequency of the antecedent among those with the illness to derive the stratum-specific etiologenetic fractions, and the overall EF can then be derived as the average of these EFs, weighted according to the distribution of the cases across the strata (cf. sect. I – 1. 2).

Community *prognosis*, regarding future levels of morbidity from a particular illness in the cared-for population, is not as much subject to having a knowledge-base from research as is clinical prognosis. To wit, the declines in the morbidity rates for degenerative cardiovascular diseases over the last two or three decades were not predicted, nor were they predictable. And while an imminent pandemic infection of H1N1 infection ('swine flu') was recently predicted, it didn't really come about.

Even though community prognosis about future morbidity from a particular illness generally is, and will be, unattainable in the practice of epidemiology, the epidemiologist's main concern nevertheless is to help bring about *reduction* in that morbidity, if at all possible; for epidemiology is, in the main, community-level preventive medicine in this meaning (cf. sect. I – 1. 2). To this end the epidemiologist may recommend, to makers of health policy, the adoption of a *regulation* to remove an etiogenetic factor from the people's environments, or mandating individuals' submission to a preventive intervention (vaccination, most notably); and/or (s)he may recommend making available a community-level *service* for people to reduce the risks for an illness or to achieve its early detection through screening. (Pursuit of early diagnosis is not preventive medicine, contrary to a common notion among epidemiologists; cf. sect. I – 1. 2.)

The epidemiologist's main line of action in the reduction of morbidity from a particular illness is, however, community-level health *education*, whether done personally or delegated – with supervision – to a health educator. Even though directed to the cared-for population at large, the aim in this is to help *individuals* in the population to take informed decisions about their own behaviors and environments (elective) relevant to their own risks for coming down with the illness (or any of the set of illnesses the risks for which would be affected). A notable consequence of this is that the knowledge-base of epidemiological preventive medicine, as it pertains to the health-education in this, is quite the same as that of clinical preventive medicine.

Of particular note in this is that insofar as risk assessment or some other care by a clinician – screening for an illness or prescription for the use of a prophylactic medication, say – may be required, the epidemiologist needs to know this and, in the health-education, encourage seeking of clinical care on particular, specified indications.

This, then, is the big picture of quintessentially 'applied' (instrumental) epidemiological research, as it here has emerged up to this point: In comparison with its clinical counterparts, the objects of community-diagnostic studies (on morbidity) are distinctly more limited in the diagnostic indicators that need to be considered; similarly, the objects of community-etiognostic studies are more limited in the inclusion and particulars of the causal histories as well as of the potential modifiers of the causal rate-ratio that are relevant to consider; and community-prognostic research is much less important, if possible at all; but, for etiologic/etiogenetic research on behavioral and environmental factors the objects of study are quite the same as they are for clinical preventive medicine.

Rather than illness-preventing interventions (artificial, such as vaccinations), preventive medicine is principally promotion of avoidance of behaviors and environments that are naturally occurring and causing illness. Experimental study of this naturally occurring causation generally is quite impractical. Therefore, the scientific knowledge-base of preventive medicine, epidemiological as well as clinical, generally is derived from *non-experimental etiogenetic/etiognostic* research.

On the other hand, though, when at issue is not change in behavior or environment but adoption of the use of a potentially preventive artifact – use of a vaccine or a chemopreventive, say – experimentation analogous to therapeutic clinical trials – the use of a *prevention trial* – is feasible. (Preventive and other clinical interventions are artificial changes in constitution; cf. 'Intervention' in sect. I – 1.2.)

In all of this I use the terms 'prevention' and 'preventive' – and address the concepts to which I take them to refer – in the framework of traditional – and still appropriate – medical terms and concepts (set forth in sect. I – 1. 2). Epidemiologists, however, have a propensity to think that only their practice – and none of that of clinicians – is preventive medicine. This leads to a tendency to enlarge the concept of prevention in healthcare. Thus, the I.E.A. dictionary says that "The concept of *prevention* is best defined in the context of *levels* of prevention, traditionally [*sic*] called, primary, secondary, and tertiary prevention. Other levels (primordial prevention, quaternary prevention) are also used." It proceeds to define all five of these. (Cf. 'Prevention' in sect. II – 2.)

'Clinical epidemiology' is not epidemiology [16]. The I.E.A. dictionary defines it as "The application of epidemiological knowledge, reasoning, and methods to study clinical issues and to improve clinical care." Health services research it defines as "The integration of knowledge from clinical, epidemiological, sociological, economic, management, and other sciences in the study of the organization, functioning, and performance of health services," while a tenable conception of this 'research' is that it actually is mere fact-finding about the occurrence (particularistic) of phenomena of healthcare – for evaluation of it, and this in terms of processes rather than outcomes [40].

II – 2. INTRODUCTORY TERMS AND CONCEPTS

The terms and concepts addressed in sections I – 1. 2, I – 2. 2, and I – 3. 2 above, are subject to criticism by academic physicians, philosophers of science, and statisticians, respectively, more than by epidemiological researchers. By contrast, the terms and concepts in this section – and in sections II – 3-4 and III – 2-4 – are, principally, for epidemiological researchers themselves to weigh and consider (cf. Preface). As in those sections above, an asterisk (*) attached to a term indicates its inclusion in the I.E.A. dictionary [4].

Analytic epidemiology* – See 'Analytic versus descriptive epidemiology.'

Analytic versus descriptive epidemiology* – The duality in etiogenetic research constituted by hypothesis-testing as distinct from hypothesis-generation and, specifically, with the idea that the unit of observation in the former is an individual, in the latter a population (large).

Note 1: In the framework of these conceptions, analytic studies are epitomized by 'cohort' and 'case-control' studies; and an example of descriptive epidemiology has been comparison between Jewish and Gentile women in respect to incidence of (the detection of) cervical cancer, leading to the hypothesis that lack of circumcision of a woman's sexual partner(s) is etiogenetic to cervical cancer.

Note 2: This duality is conceptually untenable. Those 'analytic' studies are commonly sources of etiogenetic hypotheses; and population units of observation have been deployed in hypothesis testing – regarding screening for cervical cancer, and in the famous Seven Countries Study, for example.

Note 3: This duality is linguistically untenable besides. In the 'analytic' studies – and indeed in all research – the propositions and judgments are *synthetic* rather than analytic (cf. 'Analysis and synthesis' in sect. I – 2. 2). And they too are *descriptive* of experience, even if in such a way as is judged to serve causal inference.

Note 4: Whereas the 'analytic' versus 'descriptive' duality within etiogenetic research is untenable both conceptually and linguistically, a somewhat related duality of fundamental importance is that constituted by *causal* and acausal/*descriptive* epidemiological research. While both of these inescapably are descriptive of experience, there is a profound distinction in the purpose – and consequently in the nature – of the experience being described. Within causal epidemiological research,

O. S. Miettinen, *Epidemiological Research: Terms and Concepts*,   73
DOI 10.1007/978-94-007-1171-6_5, © Springer Science+Business Media B.V. 2011

an important duality is constituted by etiogenetic and intervention studies [9], while in the descriptive research there is the ('applied') duality constituted by studies for community diagnosis and prognosis (cf. sect. II – 1).

Dependent parameter – See 'Independent parameter' (Note 2).

*Descriptive epidemiology** – See 'Analytic versus descriptive epidemiology.'

Design versus analysis – In the theory of epidemiological research at present, the perceived overarching duality: design – for data collection – as distinct from analysis – of the collected data. Thus, an authoritative article at the dawn of modern epidemiology – in the research meaning of 'epidemiology' – addressed "design and analysis of studies" [2]. At present, this duality is manifest in both the teaching and the practice of epidemiological research: design expertise is seen to be in the purview of 'epidemiologists,' analysis expertise in that of 'biostatisticians' – the two commonly cohabiting a department of 'epidemiology and biostatistics.'

Note 1: The overarching duality in the theory of epidemiological research should be understood to be that constituted by *ontic* theory on one side and *epistemic* theory on the other side: it is one thing to master the theory that guides the design of *objects* of epidemiological research, of developing plans for *what* to study; and it is quite another thing to master the theory that guides the design of *methods* of such research, of developing plans for *how* to study the designed objects of study (generally occurrence relations). Object design should be understood to be a prerequisite for meaningful methods design, methods of study being the means to study the preset object of study. Yet, remarkably, even the very concept of objects design remains absent from textbooks of epidemiological research; and the I.E.A. dictionary [4] defines study design in what appear to be singularly methodologic terms – as "The 'architecture' of a study: its structure, specific details of the studied population, time frame, method, and procedures, including ethical considerations, all of which should be explicitly stated in a research protocol." (Cf. 'Study design' in sect. II – 4.)

Note 2: Epidemiological research being concerned with *frequency* of occurrence (of phenomena of health), its objects are *statistical* in form (while medical in substance). An epidemiological researcher therefore needs to be statistically self-sufficient (apart from occasional needs to consult a statistician; cf. sect. I – 3. 1), able to design the statistical form of the object of study all the way to the particulars of the regression model to be fitted to the data that will be collected. With such completeness of object design, 'data analysis' is a piece of trivia (given the availability of modern computer software systems for this). On the other hand, thinking of 'data analysis' as a topic unto itself, not governed by object design, is tantamount to the fallacy that data 'speak' to a researcher in a meaningful way even when the researcher has not developed and implemented a closely-reasoned plan of how to 'interrogate' Nature.

Note 3: An epidemiological researcher may very well be a *statistician*. In fact, it is easier for a statistician to learn the requisite subject-matter than it is for a physician to learn the requisite statistics. For, the requisite body of statistical knowledge is quite extensive and in some respects challenging to learn, while the subject-matter knowledge for a given line of research, at the relevant depth, needs to be acquired ad hoc even by a physician and can be acquired by a statistician almost as readily.

Epidemiologic – If distinguished from 'epidemiological,' this word might denote the quality of having to do with epidemiology (as distinct from being in the nature of epidemiology).

Note: This restricted meaning is the one intended throughout this dictionary.

*Epidemiological** – If distinguished from 'epidemiologic,' this word might denote the quality of being in the nature (inherent) of epidemiology (as distinct from having to do with epidemiology).

Note: This restricted meaning is the one intended throughout this dictionary.

*Epidemiological research** – Research intended to advance, potentially at least, epidemiology (practice of it; [16]). (Cf. 'Clinical study,' Note 3, in sect. III – 2.)

Note 1: Substantively speaking, epidemiological research is about rates of the occurrence of health outcomes, but statistically speaking it is about the mean of a dependent random variate (Y, usually Bernoulli-distributed); and while epidemiological research substantively is about the occurrence of the outcome as a (joint) function of its determinants, statistically studied is the mean of Y as a (joint) function of a set of independent variates (Xs) based on the determinants. (Cf. 'Occurrence relation.')

Note 2: Epidemiological research addresses (the frequency of) the occurrence of a phenomenon (event or state) of health in a (particular type of) *human* population. (See 'Research' in sect. I – 2. 2.)

Note 3: The concept of human *population* in the objects of epidemiological research is different from that in clinical research. The meaning of 'population' here is that of a (sub)population of a notional community, of people satisfying a defined (a particular type of) state of being. It thus is an open – *dynamic* – population, not a cohort (cf. 'Dynamic population' and 'Cohort' in sect. II – 4). As at issue is research (scientific), the definitional particulars of populations are abstract (with no role for proper names in the objects of study).

Note 4: Epidemiological research, as it is here defined, can be said to be population-oriented medical research – inherently 'applied' (by the implication of 'medical'), quintessentially 'applied' when directed to the advancement of the knowledge-base of population/community medicine (epidemiology in this meaning of the term). (Cf. Preface and sect. II – 1.)

Note 5: Epidemiological research does not define epidemiology as a science, as it has no unique 'material object' (different from, e.g., neurology and cardiology in the science meanings of these terms). Various medical sciences involve epidemiological objects – such 'formal objects' – of study (akin to, e.g, morphological objects of study). (Cf. Preface and sect. I – 2. 1.)

Note 6: An epidemiological study need not be scientific, a piece of research; it can be a project of (mere) fact-finding as an element in practice. (Cf. 'Study' in sect. I – 1. 2.)

Note 7: Epidemiological research is *not epidemiology* but, instead, research *for* epidemiology (just as clinical research is not clinical medicine but, instead, research *for* clinical medicine; cf. sect. I – 1. 1, 'Medicine' in sect. I – 1. 2, and 'Epidemiology' below).

*Epidemiologist** – A physician who practices community medicine, that is, a physician whose (single) client is a 'community' – a defined population – as a whole.

Note 1: In recent decades, 'epidemiologist' has come to denote, also, a person – quite possibly not a physician – conducting, or otherwise professionally concerned with, epidemiological research and/or meta-epidemiological clinical research.

Note 2: In contrast to this expansion of the concept of epidemiologist, conduct of, or other concern with, clinical research (that of 'trialists,' say) has not become definitional to *clinician* (nor is a scholar in the field of music by definition a musician).

Epidemiologist vis-à-vis statistician – See 'Design versus analysis.'

*Epidemiology** – Community medicine (cf. sect. I – 1. 1 and 'Medicine' in sect. I – 1. 2).

Note 1: In recent decades, epidemiological research has become an added denotation of 'epidemiology' – even as clinical research has not become an added denotation of 'clinical medicine.' (Cf. 'Epidemiologist' above.)

Note 2: Even if epidemiological research is (seen to be) epidemiology, theory of epidemiological research is not epidemiology (just as, say, theory of chess is not chess and theory of gambling is not gambling).

*Exposure** – See section I – 1. 2.

*Factor** – See section I – 1. 2.

*False negative/positive** – See section I – 1. 2.

Genetics vis-à-vis epidemiology – Genetical and epidemiological research have areas of overlap. For one, some illnesses are, in their definitions, genetic anomalies (e.g., trisomy 21). Study of the occurrence of these illnesses is as much epidemiological as it is genetical, including occurrence-based study of the etiogenesis of them; it is as much *genetical epidemiology* as it is *epidemiological genetics*. For another, study of genetic factors in the etiogenesis of illnesses, as prognostic markers, or as modifiers of the effects of interventions also is as much genetical epidemiology as it is epidemiological genetics.

Note 1: In epidemiological research one does not study determinants of the occurrence of illness, genetic or other; one studies, instead, the occurrence of illness – the frequency of this – *in relation to* – as a function of – the determinants of this. Study of the nature of genetic phenomena (states and events) is in the domain of genetics alone, extrinsic to epidemiology.

Note 2: *Population genetics* is genetics and not epidemiology, except when at issue is the occurrence of a genetic anomaly that is definitional to an illness (cf. above).

Health services research* – "The integration of knowledge from clinical, epidemiological, sociological, economic, management, and other sciences in the study of the organization, functioning, and performance of health services. . . . The aim of health services research is evaluation; several components of evaluative health services research are distinguished, namely: 1. Evaluation of *structure*, . . . 2. . . . *process*, . . . 3. . . . *output*, . . . 4. . . . *outcome*, concerned with the results – i.e., whether persons using health services experience measurable benefits, such as improved survival or reduced disability" [4].

Note 1: In part due to its pleonastic nature (nothing uncommon in the I.E.A. dictionary), this definition poses a hermeneutical challenge. Even though the term involves the word "research," the definition does not specify research – or study – as the concept's (obvious) proximal genus, and the object of this research as the specific difference (cf. 'Concept' in sect. I – 2. 2). Instead, quite incongruously with the term, the proximal genus is said to be "integration," and the specific difference then is a matter of what is integrated in what context – namely "knowledge" (*sic*) from a variety of disciplines, and this in the context of studying certain aspects of "health services."

Note 2: Presumably intended was this: Health services research is research on (the various aspects of) *quality* of health services (for evaluation of the quality). A prime example – generic – of this research is study of the (rate of) occurrence of a given type of malpractice in a particular type of situation in the practice of medicine.

Note 3: It is commonplace to distinguish between quality and *cost* of healthcare, where meant by cost is not the inherent cost of a given type of care (in neonatal intensive-care units, say) but that to which efforts of cost-containment are directed: cost arising from waste, from inefficient practices. Cost in this meaning is not distinct from, but an aspect of, the quality of healthcare: at issue is (wanting) *economic quality*, as distinct from medical quality.

Note 4: Assessment of the quality of a given element of healthcare (e.g., diagnostic testing in the context of a given complaint in the patient presentation) presupposes an agreed-upon *scale* (ordinal) of quality, anchored to definition of good – normative – care. Data on the frequencies of particular degrees of deviation from a particular norm constitute the requisite input to evaluative judgments about the element of care at issue (cf. 'Evaluation' in sect. I – 1. 2.)

Note 5: Acquisition of data for evaluative judgments about healthcare is *not research*: rather than scientific inquiry (about the abstract), it is mere fact-finding (about the particularistic) – even if very important at that.

Note 6: 'Health services' is a misnomer for healthcare, just as 'research' is a misnomer for particularistic inquiries. (Cf. 'Health services' in sect. I – 1. 2 and 'Research' in sect. I – 2. 2.)

Note 7: "Whether persons using health services experience … improved survival and reduced disability" or whatever other "benefits" are questions of actual research, most notably by RCTs, and not of fact-finding for evaluation of quality of healthcare. (Cf. 'Outcomes research' in sect. III – 2.)

*Hypothesis** – In epidemiological research, typically, a conjecture about an etiogenetic effect/role of an antecedent of an illness (when contrasting the antecedent with its defined alternative). (Cf. 'Hypothesis' in sect. I – 2. 2 and I – 3. 2, and 'Null hypothesis' below.)

Hypothesis testing – The conduct of a study intended to serve updating of the degree of credibility/plausibility accorded to a hypothesis. (See 'Causal inference' and 'Causal criteria/considerations.')

Note 1: Just as any other type of testing – glucose-tolerance testing, say – this hypothesis-testing ends with the attainment of its evidentiary result: just as knowing – diagnosis – about the presence/absence of Type II diabetes is a matter separate from (and subsequent to) the GTT, so *inference* about the correctness/incorrectness of an etiogenetic hypothesis is *not part of the testing* of the hypothesis. Inference about the correctness/incorrectness of the hypothesis is *not* a proper concern for the hypothesis-testing investigators; it is a concern of the relevant scientific community. (Cf. Note 3 under 'Study' in sect. I – 2.2.)

Note 2: The testing actually is not directly about the correctness/incorrectness of the hypothesis itself but, instead, about that of the corresponding 'null hypothesis' of *no effect*, and the test's result (evidentiary) pertains in direct terms to something different even from this: it pertains to the corresponding statistical 'null hypothesis' of *no association* – in such terms as the association (descriptive) got to be defined by the study's object and methods designs (and the execution of the latter).

Note 3: For the substantive and statistical 'null hypotheses' to cohere, required is all of the following: The conditioning of the comparative parameter (rate ratio) according to the (form of the) designed theoretical occurrence relation must fully account for the alternative to causality (potential confounding, i.e.); the translation of this theoretical occurrence relation into its operational counterpart must not compromise the meaning of the designed theoretical occurrence relation (notably the rate-ratio's intended conditionality on a particular set of potential confounders); and the methods design (and execution) must assure freedom from descriptive bias in the result of the study (selection and documentation bias; sect. II – 4).

Note 4: For any intended-to-be hypothesis-testing to actually be such testing, the study must have a virtue beyond freedom from bias: it must have at least a modicum of propensity to produce evidence against the substantive 'null hypothesis' insofar as this indeed is incorrect. This means, in the context of whatever may be the efficiency and size of the study, that the etiogenetic histories need to address the etiogenetically relevant span of time (on the scale of etiogenetic time). This is particularly important to appreciate in studies to test hypotheses about the etiogenesis of a cancer (as the initiation of a cancer readily is decades in the past when viewed from the vantage of the time of its first overt manifestation). *Pseudo-testing* of these hypotheses is, unfortunately, not uncommon at present, still.

*Independence** – Lack of association (theoretical) between an outcome and a potential determinant of (the rate of) its occurrence; also: among causal determinants, absence of synergism, antagonism, and interaction.

Independent parameter – In a regression model, any particular one of the regression coefficients (incl. the intercept).

   Note 1: This term is a here-suggested neologism, patterned after 'independent variate' (sect. I – 3. 2). Those coefficients are treated as constants of Nature (for the domain of the model, conditionally on the other independent variates involved in the model).

   Note 2: Correspondingly, the mean of the dependent variate, or a transform of this, is the *dependent parameter* in the framework of a regression model; its value depends on the independent variates and parameters.

*Indicator variate** – A variate with 0 and 1 as its (only) realizations, with realization 1 indicating something particular. (Examples: $Y = 1$ indicating membership in the case series of person-moments and $X_1 = 1$ indicating index category of the etiogenetic determinant in an etiogenetic study – in the logistic model for the object of study.)

*Induction period** – See section I – 1. 2.

*Latency period** – See section I – 1. 2.

*Null hypothesis** – The denial of a hypothesis (in epidemiology, typically, about etiogenesis). The denial inherently pertains to all subdomains of the referent domain of the hypothesis.

   Note: In science (epidemiological or whatever), all effects – and descriptive differences also – are supposed to be regarded as being nil until there is good reason to think otherwise. This is the backdrop for adducing a hypothesis – an inspired idea (conducive to insomnia in the one who experiences the inspiration. The genesis of a hypothesis is, to one extent or another, a 'flash of genius'). Thus, the denial of a hypothesis is *not a hypothesis*; it is merely the expected stance until there is adequate reason to regard the hypothesis as being true, as having become a piece of scientific knowledge. (Cf. 'Hypothesis' in sect. I – 2. 2.)

*Prevention/preventive** – See section II – 1 and 'Intervention' in section I – 1. 2.

   Note: The I.E.A. dictionary defines five types/levels of prevention – from "primordial" to "quaternary" – as though curative medicine were subsumed under preventive medicine. (Cf. 'Curative' in sect. I – 1. 2.)

Quantitative research – Statistical research.

Note: This term originates from statistics and is applied, in statistical science, to hypothesis-testing as well as to quantification (of the magnitudes of parameters in the objects of studies). Substantively, however, only research for quantification/estimation is quantitative.

*Research design** – See 'Study design' (Note 3).

*Screening** – See section I – 1. 2.

*Study design** – The structure of an epidemiological study in its ad-hoc particulars (substantive, given its a-priori generic structure) together with the way in which this structure and substantive content were/are to be produced in the process of the study. (See Note 2 under 'Analysis and synthesis' in sect. I – 2. 2.)

Note 1: The a-priori generic structure of an epidemiological study, so long as it is logically admissible, is dictated by the generic nature of the *object* of study. The ad-hoc particulars – substantive – in the framework of this structure also are dictated by the object design for the study, but only in conceptual terms. (Cf. 'Etiologic study' in sect. II – 4 and 'Intervention study' in sect. III – 4.) The study's *methods design* specifies only the operationalizations of the (conceptual) elements in the structure, as well as the way in which this structure and substantive content were/are to come about (cf. 'Design' in sect. II – 4).

Note 2: As is thus evident, the principal components of epidemiological study design could be taken to be the study's object design and its methods design, with the latter subordinate to the former; but perhaps a preferable view is that deliberate object design is a necessary precursor – a prerequisite – for study design in the merely epistemic meaning of rational methods design.

Note 3: The *term* 'study design' in epidemiological contexts has recently, quite commonly (incl. in the I.E.A. dictionary), been discarded in preference to 'research design.' Yet, at issue is design of only a piece of research, rather than the entirety of studies on the object of study at issue.

Note 4: For further conceptual orientation to study design, see 'Design and analysis.'

*Survey** – In community medicine, acquisition of information about the cared-for population by means of drawing a sample of the population (of person-moments in it), ascertaining the information/facts on the instances in the sample, and generalizing from this to the population (the 'target population').

Note: Such particularistic inquiry is *not research* (see sect. I – 2. 2).

Theory – Concerning epidemiological (or meta-epidemiological clinical) research at large, the general concepts, principles, and terminology of this (distinct from ones specific to particular topics of subject-matter).

Note 1: This book obviously is about the theory of epidemiological and meta-epidemiological clinical research in respect to *concepts* of these, and also about their associated English-language *terms* (this is the sequence of these two in their development, in contrast to their sequence in a dictionary); and just as obviously, this book, like the I.E.A. dictionary, is preparatory to expositions of *principles* of these lines of research.

Note 2: Once well-grounded on the concepts (and terms) – tenable concepts (and terms) – of these lines of research, one's 'natural logic' (distinct from 'acquired, scientific logic') becomes quite a good guide to the principles of the research. Acquisition of the requisite, logically tenable concepts goes a long way in preparing a student for adopting the proper principles for the research. In fact, principles are critically involved in the genesis of many of the concepts, including absolutely central ones such as that of *the* etiologic study (as the outgrowth of the 'cohort' and 'case-control' studies).

Note 3: The I.E.A. dictionary [4] asserts that the theory of epidemiological research addresses (specifically and solely) "how to study" – methods of epidemiologic research, that is. But the theory of *methods* design for epidemiological research – epistemic – is subordinate to the ontic theory of the design of *objects* of epidemiological research (both of which rest on critically adopted concepts of epidemiological research).

Note 4: Theory of epidemiological research is first – orientationally – *general theory*, addressing the concepts and principles of the research, without reference to any particular area of subject-matter. This book is about general theory of epidemiological – and meta-epidemiological clinical – research in respect to the concepts the research. Concepts of the practice of epidemiology are addressed only insofar as they bear on understanding those of the research.

*Theory of epidemiology** – Concepts, principles, and terminology of epidemiology (of the practice of community medicine); in particular, general concepts and principles, and corresponding terms across particular topics of subject-matter.

Note 1: Theory of community medicine is one of the two principal components of *theory of medicine* (the other one being theory of clinical medicine).

Note 2: If the concept of epidemiology is taken to subsume epidemiological research (while no-one takes clinical research to be clinical medicine), then theory of epidemiological research is subsumed by that of epidemiology. (Cf. 'Epidemiologist' and 'Epidemiology.')

II – 3. TERMS AND CONCEPTS OF OBJECTS OF STUDY

See note opening section II – 2.

Administrative – Concerning the object of an epidemiological study, the quality of having to do with care providers' (professional) behavior rather than truths about Nature. (Cf. 'Health services research' in sect. II – 2.)

Note 1: Administrative epidemiological studies are not research (inherently scientific); they are matters of fact-finding for a particularistic purpose – most notably for quality-assurance and/or cost-containment in a system of healthcare.

Note 2: Even though not scientific, administrative epidemiological studies are of great importance, commonly more consequential than epidemiological studies of the scientific sort; they always have immediate (if only local) implications, in principle at least.

Admissibility – Concerning the object of an epidemiological study (scientific), the quality of being formally – logically – correct. (See 'Quality of study object[s].')

*Antagonism** – The interrelation between two causes in which one inhibits (to whatever extent) the effect of the other. (Cf. 'Synergism.')

*Association** – The relation of an outcome to an antecedent such that the outcome's rate of occurrence has the antecedent as a determinant (in a theoretical association); also: this pattern in the study experience (in an empirical association; cf. sect. II – 4).

Category (synonyms: class, division) – See section I – 2. 2.

Note: Remarkably, a category/range of age is quite routinely misnomered as 'age group' in epidemiologic writings, while 'gender group' is not a term used in reference to a category of gender. (See 'Group.')

Causal contrast – Contrast (as to the outcome's rate of occurrence) between the cause (potential) at issue and its particular alternative (which commonly is not simply absence of the cause). (Examples: regular heavy consumption of alcohol vs. no consumption of alcohol with the energy-equivalent added intake of, specifically,

O. S. Miettinen, *Epidemiological Research: Terms and Concepts,*
DOI 10.1007/978-94-007-1171-6_6, © Springer Science+Business Media B.V. 2011

complex carbohydrates, say; regular engagement in jogging or similar exercise vs. sedentary life-style but with energy-intake correspondingly lower while similar in composition; regular use of a particular analgesic vs. regular use of a particular other analgesic; and a given type of preventive intervention vs. a particular alternative type of preventive care – instead of contrasting the former with 'usual care,' which is an undefined melange of particulars.)

Note 1: The causal contrast – cause versus its alternative – does not have as its referent instances that differ in this respect (cause present in some, the alternative in others). Instead, the contrast has to do with all of the instances of the study domain (and study base) in the same way: the contrast is between all instances of the domain with the cause present (hypothetically) versus all of them with the alternative present (hypothetically). The contrast has to do with two mutually exclusive possibilities in each instance of the study domain, at least one of them a hypothetical (counterfactual).

Note 2: While most of physics can be thought in merely descriptive, acausal terms (commonly mathematically expressed), and while philosophers may argue about the admissibility/reality of the very concept of causality (sect. I – 2. 2), medicine (incl. epidemiology) without this concept would be as passive about human health as astrophysics and cosmology are about the goings-on in the extraterrestrial cosmos.

Causal determinant – In a causality-oriented epidemiological study (etiogenetic or interventive), the determinant (potential at least, of the outcome's occurrence) that is of focal concern. (The cause – potential at least – at issue is a particular category of this determinant, while the alternative is another particular category of it.) (Cf. "Risk factor.')

Note: It is convenient to use the term 'causal determinant' even when the existence of the causality remains a mere possibility (hypothesis). The term can be taken to mean, merely, a person-characterizer with at least the potential of being a causal determinant (according to the hypothesis).

Causal rate-ratio – The object of an etiogenetic study.

Note 1: As causation is not a phenomenon (but, instead, an aprioristic noumenon; cf. sect. I – 2. 2), study of it requires definition of a phenomenal pattern of the occurrence of the illness at issue (in the abstract) such that this pattern implies a *descriptive RR* deemed to be a manifestation (solely, or nearly so) of the magnitude of the causal RR of interest; it requires design of (the form of) an *occurrence relation* (descriptive) such that it implies what the manifestation of the causal RR is taken to be – in the referent *domain* of that relation/function. Design of the object (causal RR) of an etiogenetic study requires design of such an occurrence relation (as to its form and domain).

Note 2: An etiogenetic *hypothesis* implies that the causal RR (contrasting the cause with its alternative) is greater than unity – in a particular, specified domain. For testing such a hypothesis, the designed occurrence relation need not have but one parameter representing (what is presumed to be) the causal RR, this as the measure of the causal association (between the outcome and the particular etiogenetic determinant of the rate of its occurrence).

Note 3: The hypothesis means nothing more than (the conjecture) that the causal null state does not obtain; that is, that causal RR = 1 does not obtain for all sub-domains of the occurrence relation's domain. In particular, it does not mean (the conjecture) that the (causal) RR has some particular, singular value (unknown) in its hypothesized range (RR > 1) in all subdomains of the domain (abstract) at issue (just as it would have in the null state of Nature).

Note 4: As a simple – quite simplistic but instructive – example, designed for a study to test an etiogenetic *hypothesis* could be this (statistical form of the) occurrence relation for a particular, defined domain (abstract):

$$\log(\mathrm{ID}') = \sum_0^4 B_i X_i,$$

where

ID$'$ is the numerical value, as defined, of the outcome event's incidence density (ID),

$X_0 = 1$,

X_1 is the defined, single variate (numerical) representing age (at the time of outcome, the event's occurrence/non-occurrence, in the domain),

X_2 is the defined gender variate (indicator of a particular one of the two genders),

X_3 is indicator of positive history, as defined, about the potential cause, and

X_4 is indicator of history that is neither positive (cause present) nor negative (alternative present).

This design for the occurrence relation relevant for the testing of the hypothesis implies the judgment that $B_3 > 0$ corresponds to the etiogenetic hypothesis, $B_3 = 0$ to the null state, B_3 representing the logarithm of the ID ratio – descriptive – for the causal contrast. This design for the occurrence relation implies the judgment that the descriptive ID ratio, in the domain at issue, represents the causal ID ratio when conditional on (only) age and gender (and with age accounted for in that simple, log-linear way).

Note 5: Continuing with that simple example, if the hypothesis already has become a matter of (not merely someone's conjecture but) actual knowledge (among experts) and *quantification* of the effect's magnitude has become the scientific concern, the designed occurrence relation – defining the way the investigators think about the causal RR's magnitude (unknown) – could be this:

$$\log(\mathrm{ID}') = \sum_0^6 B_i X_i,$$

where

ID$'$ and X_0 through X_4 are as in Note 4 above,

X_5 is $X_1 X_3$, and

X_6 is $X_2 X_3$.

Implied by this is the judgment that, contrasting the positive history with the negative history, the difference in $\log(\text{ID}') - B_3 + B_5X_1 + B_6X_2$ – translates into the causal RR as

$$\text{IDR} = \exp(B_3 + B_5X_1 + B_6X_2),$$

IDR being the incidence-density ratio in the contrasting of the index history with the reference history in the domain at issue.

Note 6: Why, one might ask, is it the rate *ratio* rather than the corresponding rate difference that is to be the object of an etiogenetic study? One argument to this effect has to do with imagining that causation actually is a phenomenon, observable and (thereby) documentable. If this were the case, the questions would be these: Of the cases of the outcome event (change) occurring in the domain at issue with the potential cause at issue an antecedent, are any of them caused by this antecedent? and if so, what *proportion* of the cases with the antecedent? That orientational question corresponds, quite interchangeably, to asking whether the causal rate-ratio equals unity and whether the causal rate difference equals zero (in the domain at issue); but that question about the magnitude of that proportion is one about the etiogenetic *proportion* among the cases of the outcome with the antecedent such that the antecedent is causal to the outcome; and the magnitude of that proportion is determined by the causal rate *ratio*, not the rate difference, in the domain at issue. (Cf. 'Etiogenetic proportion' in sect. I – 1. 2.)

Causal versus descriptive research – See 'Analytic versus descriptive epidemiology,' Note 4, in section II – 2.

*Causation** – A cause producing its effect (as a sufficient cause or by completing a sufficient cause). (Cf. 'Preventive' under 'Intervention' in section I – 1. 2.)

Cause – See 'Causal contrast' and 'Sufficient cause.'

Characteristic – In the occurrence relation constituting or defining the object of an epidemiological study, a particular category or level of a person-characterizer.

Characterizer – In the occurrence relation constituting or defining the object of an epidemiological study, an aspect of persons in terms of which a given determinant (of the rate of the outcome's occurrence) is defined; it is this dimension of characterization, distinct from a realization of it as a particular characteristic of a person (specific to a particular moment in time, perhaps). (Example: age as a dimension in which a person, at a particular moment in time, may be characterized – as to what the age at that moment happens to be.)

Note: Person-characterizers in the objects of epidemiological studies fall in the broadest categories of constitutional (congenital and acquired), behavioral, and environmental (a person's environment, too, being a characterizer of him/her).

*Class** (synonyms: category, division) – See 'Category.'

Comparative parameter – The object of a causal epidemiological study (etio-genetic/etiognostic or intervention-prognostic) as a measure of the magnitude of the effect; also: a measure of the 'strength' of an acausal association (for a comparison of a rate between the two genders, say).

Note 1: The object of any causal study is comparative because the very concept of cause involves its comparison with its alternative. (Cf. 'Causal contrast.')

Note 2: The comparative parameter is, inherently, different between an etio-logic/etiogenetic study and an intervention study (rate ratio and rate difference, respectively).

Note 3: Actually the object in causal studies is descriptive – a descriptive coun-terpart of the causal measure, though with such conditionality as is judged necessary for causal inference. (Cf. Note 1 under 'Causal rate-ratio.')

Credibility (synonym: plausibility) – Concerning an idea, the degree – subjective – of its verisimilitude.

*Cross-sectional** (synonym: synchronic; antonyms: longitudinal, diachronic) – Concerning the occurrence relation defining the object of an etiogenetic study, the quality that the temporal referent of the (potentially) causal determinant (of the rate of the outcome's occurrence) is not the actual range of etiogenetically relevant time (retrospective, with T_0 the time of outcome), nor even a segment of this; that it is, instead, reduced (by object design) to a mere point in time and, specifically, to the point coincident with the outcome (its occurrence/non-occurrence). (Cf. Note 9 under 'Time.')

Dependent parameter – See 'Independent parameter' (Note 2) in section II – 2.

*Dichotomous** – Concerning an element in the object of study, the quality of being constituted by (only) two categories. (Cf. 'Trichotomous' and 'Polytomous.')

Note: A dichotomy is statistically represented by an indicator (0, 1) variate.

Domain – Concerning the object of an epidemiological study (scientific), the cate-gory (of the abstract) that is its referent. (Example: For a study about the etiogenesis of a cancer by paucity/deficiency of a particular micro-nutrient in the diet, the domain should perhaps be characterized by suitably advanced age – for the occur-rence to be common-enough for serious concern and for the etiogenetic histories to be longitudinal/diachronic enough.)

*Effect** – Concerning a cause, the change produced by its being present (in lieu of its alternative) – in epidemiology, mainly, the increase in the level of morbidity from an illness.

Note: The I.E.A. dictionary says, under 'Effect,' this: "The result of a cause. In epidemiology, frequently a synonym for effect measure." But where the concept of effect is equated with any measure of it, the researchers are using the word 'effect' in the loose meaning that prevails in statistics. (In clinical medicine, the concept of, say, glucose intolerance is not equated with any particular measure of it.) (See 'Effect measure.')

*Effect measure** – Concerning a comparative parameter for a causal contrast, its magnitude's deviation from its null value (representing no effect).

Note 1: In an etiogenetic study the comparative parameter is rate ratio (contrasting the causal determinant's index – causal – category against its reference – alternative – category), conditional on certain potential confounders; and the effect measure is the extent to which this RR exceeds unity.

Note 2: This effect measure (RR – 1) is theoretical – a parameter – in the object of a study, empirical as the result of a study and also as the result of inference (from all studies on it).

*Effect modification** – Concerning an effect measure, its magnitude's dependence on one or more characterizers of persons.

Estimation – See section I – 1. 2.

Note: In epidemiological research, estimation is inference in the face of evidence from a quantification (rather than hypothesis-testing) study. Production of an empirical value for a parameter is not estimation (cf. sect. I – 3. 2).

*Etiogenesis/etiognosis/etiology** – See section I – 1. 2.

Etiologic/etiogenetic time – See 'Time' (Note 9).

*Exposure** – In the object of an etiogenetic study, the index category of the causal determinant.

Note 1: This term, while in ubiquitous use in writings about epidemiological research at present, is a misnomer when used in this meaning. One is not really 'exposed' to one's own constitutional or behavioral characteristics. Only in reference to environmental characteristics is the word really apposite. (Cf. sect. I – 1. 2.)

Note 2: According to the I.E.A. dictionary [4], exposure is, in one – the first one – of the meanings of the word, "The variable whose causal effect is to be estimated." But: In science, different from statistics, there are no non-causal effects (cf. 'Effect' in sect. I – 3. 2); in epidemiological research there is hypothesis-testing in addition to – and always before – 'estimation' (quantification); and a sharp distinction is to be made between substantive characterizers of persons (as to exposure or whatever) and the statistical (numerical) variates adopted ad hoc to represent these.

*Factor** – See section I – 1. 2.

*Index category** – See 'Index and reference categories.'

Index and reference categories – In a causal determinant, the categories representing the cause and its alternative, respectively [12]. (Cf. 'Causal determinant.')

Note 1: In general English, one of the meanings of 'index' has to do with pointing (as in 'index finger'); and pointing is involved in the present context. In a causal determinant, the two categories involved in a causal contrast are not viewed symmetrically, in a similar way; instead, attention is focused – quite pointedly – on the category constituting the cause, even if not as a category per se but only as a category of interest when occurring in lieu of its particular alternative (rather than, merely, in lieu of its absence). While the cause is the index category in this meaning of 'index,' the alternative is the corresponding reference category in the same sense as a reference laboratory completes the meaning of the results from a laboratory of focal (local) interest.

Note 2: For the reference category, the term 'referent' is a (not uncommon) misnomer. The reference category is not that to which a 'cause' refers; it is part of the very concept of cause, in the referent domain of the causation at issue.

Indicator – See 'Risk indicator.'

Insufficient cause – See 'Sufficient cause' (Note 4).

Intervention time – See 'Time' (Note 10).

*Latency period** – See 'Time' (Note 11).

*Longitudinal** (synonym: diachronic; antonyms: cross-sectional, synchronic) – Concerning the occurrence relation defining the object of an etiogenetic study, the quality that the temporal referent of the (potentially) causal determinant (of the rate of the outcome's occurrence) is retrospective in etiogenetic time (the T_0 of which is the time of the outcome, its occurrence/non-occurrence). (Cf. Note 9 under 'Time.')

*Necessary cause** – See 'Sufficient cause' (Note 5).

*Objective** of study* – To produce evidence on (the truth about) the object of study (for inferences about the object of study, by members of the relevant scientific community).

Note 1: Some medical journals require that the Abstract or Summary of a research report state the Objective of the study. This, however, should be understood always to be that of producing evidence on (the truth about) the object of study. Instead of the Objective, the journals should require a specification of the Object of study, and not only in the report's Abstract/Summary but in its full version as well. But, most remarkably, it seems that no medical journal does this. (The journals invariably expect the report to address the study methodology – as the means to the objective of producing evidence about an unspecified object of study).

Note 2: When required to state the Objective of their study, epidemiologists commonly write that it was 'to study' whatever they did study. But studying is but the process aspect of the means to the end of producing evidence; it is not the objective to which the studying is directed.

Object of study – In epidemiological research, the occurrence relation designed (as to its form and domain) with the idea that the magnitude(s) of the parameter(s) in it would be studied (qualitatively, in hypothesis-testing, or quantitatively, for estimation). (See 'Occurrence relation' and 'Causal rate-ratio.')

Occurrence relation – The generic object of epidemiological research, specified by its form, as designed, in the context of any given study. In the context of a particular study it expresses the terms in which the investigators, upon the object-design considerations (of relevance, etc.) elect to think about a particular outcome's (rate of) occurrence within a particular domain of this occurrence, specifically as to the rate's dependence on its determinants within this domain.

Note 1: In the context of an *etiogenetic* study the domain is one of the outcome's occurrence. One of the determinants of (the rate of) the outcome's occurrence is, of course, the causal determinant at issue. Other determinants also are generally included, as potential confounders. While this is all that belongs in the occurrence relation designed to define the object of a study to test an etiogenetic hypothesis, a corresponding quantification study (in the context of a known cause) generally requires some of the causal rate-ratio's potential modifiers to be included in the occurrence relation. (Cf. 'Causal rate-ratio.')

Note 2: In the context of an etiogenetic study, the designed occurrence relation does not constitute the object of study in its entirety. Instead, the occurrence relation is designed as the necessary definition of what the causal RR is take to be about, descriptively. Thus, for a hypothesis-testing study addressing incidence of a cancer (operationally in terms of the incidence of the cancer's first rule-in diagnosis), a log-linear model for that event's incidence density is designed, with a need for an (independent) parameter representing the RR's logarithm. The rest of the linear compound defines the conditionality of this judged-to-be measure of causal association, descriptive though it is. (Cf. 'Causal rate-ratio.')

*Outcome** – If used (as is common) as a synonym for 'effect,' this term should be Ockham's-razored away from the lexicons of epidemiology. But the term is useful in the *descriptive* sense of result: the occurrence of the outcome may be studied for causal inference about these occurrences (in etiogenetic and intervention research) as well as, of course, in descriptive research. Generally, in epidemiological research, 'outcome' is the generic term for the illness whose occurrence is at issue.

*Outcomes research** – See section III – 2.

Person-characteristic – See 'Characteristic'/'Characterizer' and 'Variable.'

*Person-time** – A (very common) misnomer for population-time. (Cf. 'Time,' incl. Notes 1 and 2.)

Person-years* – See 'Time' (Note 1).

Plausibility* (synonym: credibility) – See 'Credibility' and 'Quality of study object(s).'

Polytomous* – Concerning an element in the object of study, the quality of being constituted by several (or many) categories. (Cf. 'Dichotomous' and 'Trichotomous.')
   Note 1: A polytomy is statistically represented indicator (0, 1) variates one fewer than the number of categories involved, each variate indicating a separate category.
   Note 2: At variance with this, the I.E.A. dictionary defines the 'polytomous' quality as "A categorical variable [sic] with three [sic] or more categories" – with the common failure to distinguish between phenomena and their representation by statistical variates.

Population* – See 'Cohort' and 'Dynamic population' – and also 'Group' – in section II – 4.

Population-time – See 'Time' (Note 1).

Primary objectives – The objectives that are the justification for the study (as distinct from objectives that the study justifies – as ancillary objectives). (Cf. 'Secondary objectives.')

Prospective* – See 'Time' (Notes 8, 10, and 12).

Quality of study object(s) – That which is the concern to 'optimize' – to maximize – in the design of the object(s) of a study (epidemiological). In studying the etiology/etiogenesis of an illness (which is what epidemiological research mostly is about), the quality desiderata – some of them actual requirements – in the design of the object of study (the causal rate-ratio implied by the designed occurrence relation for its designed domain) are:

1. *Admissibility* of the hypothesis. The imperatives of logic are inviolate in genuine science, and this makes a hypothesis that is in violation of scientific logic inadmissible into science. The first requirement for the admissibility of a proposition constituting a hypothesis is *objectivity* of its terms, most notably as to what the causal contrast is taken to be (qualitatively speaking). Then, the contrast's *rationality* requires not only that it be retrospective on the scale of etiogenetic time but also that both the index history and the reference history actually are imaginable for the same person. The fundamental given, with no alternative imaginable, in the context of a given individual is the particular pair of gametes from which the individual developed. This means that for a person's gender (as for XX vs. XY) and age (as of conception), no alternative is imaginable, and that, therefore, they are not admissible as hypothesized etiogenetic factors. But a given pair of gametes

does not inherently represent a particular genetic endowment: for euploidy, various types of uneuploidy are possible alternatives (as for, e.g., chromosome 21 in the etiogenesis of Down's syndrome); and by the same token, for whatever haplotype in a given gamete, mutational alternatives are well imaginable.

2. *Plausibility** of the hypothesis. Causal RR in respect to quite an implausible hypothesis is of low quality as the object of an etiogenetic study. Example of low plausibility (arguably at least): radio-frequency electromagnetic radiation (non-ionizing) from a cell phone, this in the rather recent past, as a cause of (clinical cases of) brain cancer.

3. *Relevance** of the hypothesis. If the hypothesized causation of the illness were to obtain, could knowledge of the magnitude of the causal RR lead to preventive actions and, thereby, to appreciable – cost-justifying – reduction in morbidity from the illness? Regarding a relevant hypothesis the answer to this question is affirmative: the illness is serious (incl. commonly incurable); the presence of the cause is practically recognizable and may represent substantial increase in the risk for the illness; and the cause is feasible to avoid. Examples: Genetic etiogenesis, quite broadly, may not qualify; poverty generally does not; but maternal diethyl stilbesterol use in the etiogenesis of clear-cell carcinoma of the vagina in girls does, even though the absolute risk is low.

4. *Testability* of the hypothesis. One requirement (obvious) is that the requisite conditionality of the RR for causal inference, the conditioning characterizers (of people) are to be subject to sufficiently accurate documentation (for control of confounding). Example: The hypothesis that use of aspirin in febrile illness in children is etiogenetic to Reye's syndrome was tested by exceptionally high-profile studies, with concern to address the RR conditionally on the level of fever; but documentation of this potential confounder was infeasible, mainly due to the antipyresis by the use of aspirin. This problem was a consequence of the causal contrast having been designed to involve no use of aspirin as the alternative to the use of aspirin. Had the object of study been designed to address the contrast between the use of aspirin and the use of acetaminophen, say, confounding by the indication for antipyresis would not have been a concern – and in these terms the hypothesis would have been more realistically testable. Another requirement (also obvious) is that the determinant histories are to be ascertainable with sufficient accuracy. Example: Etiogenesis of cancer from diets deficient in anti-oxidants is not testable so long as suitable records of dietary habits in childhood and early adulthood are not available for people in the sixth and later decades of age.

5. Admissibility for *quantification*. A designed object of study for quantification is in violation of the imperatives of logic if the idea is to address quantitatively the comparative parameter (RR) in reference to a contrast that lacks *specificity* (as to the relevant particulars of the index and reference histories as functions of etiogenetic time, the entirety of this); and even in reference to a suitably specific causal contrast, the objective of providing evidence for estimation is wanting in rationality if specificity in respect to notable modifiers of the effect parameter's (RR's) magnitude is wanting in the designed object of study. (A single non-null

magnitude for the causal RR is a mere phantasm as the object of estimation, for an ever-never contrast in particular.) And besides, setting out to provide for estimation before the hypothesis has matured to knowledge is a breach of scientific logic.

*Rate** – See section I – 1. 2.

*Rate ratio** – The object of study in etiogenetic research, specifically index rate (theoretical) divided by reference rate (theoretical).

*Reference category** – See 'Index and reference categories.'

Referent – Concerning a term, the concept it represents (as its denotation); also: concerning a concept, another concept constituting the context for its full meaning. (Prime example: A designed type of occurrence relation has its domain as its referent: it is in reference to this domain that the design has its meaning. Related example: A causal rate-ratio has a particular occurrence relation, for a particular domain, as its referent, as the context for the meaning of the concept at issue.)

*Relative risk** – See 'Attributable and relative risk' in section II – 4.

*Relevance** – See 'Quality of study object(s).'

*Research design** – See 'Study design' (Note 3) in section II – 2.

*Retrospective** – See 'Time' (Notes 8–10, 12).

*Risk factor** – A causal determinant of the occurrence of an adverse outcome (cf. 'Factor' in section I – 1. 2).

Risk indicator – A determinant of a rate (acausal or causal); cf. 'Indicator' in sect. I – 1. 2.

RR – Rate ratio (theoretical).

Scientific time – See 'Time' (Note 9).

Secondary objectives – Objectives that are/were not involved in the justification of the study but are/were justified by the study (for the primary objectives of it). (Cf. 'Primary objectives,' and 'Ancillary study' in sect. II – 4.)

Study design – See section II – 2.

Subdomain – A subcategory of the category constituting the study domain, specified by (realizations of) the descriptive determinants of (the rate of) the outcome's occurrence. (See 'Category.')

Note: The causal determinant in an etiogenetic or intervention-prognostic study does not specify subdomains of the study (object's) domain due to the very nature of causality. (Cf. 'Causal contrast.')

*Sufficient cause** – A cause that, in the context of survival-based opportunity for the effect/change at issue, unconditionally/ineluctably produces it.

Note 1: Any sufficient cause of a cancer is a sufficient cause of an overt case of the cancer only in the context of the person surviving the entire period from the cancer's inception to its clinical manifestation, without the cancer being cured in its preclinical stages. As in this example, a sufficient cause has its *immediate* effect (here bringing about inception of cancer) unconditionally, its *delayed* effect (here bringing about overt cancer) conditionally only.

Note 2: A *proximate* sufficient cause of an overt case of an infectious disease is constituted by effective exposure to the agent in conjunction with susceptibility to it, in the context of survival through the incubation period. (Cf. 'Agent' in sect. I – 1. 2.)

Note 3: A sufficient cause of a sufficient cause of an illness is a sufficient cause of the illness.

Note 4: Any *insufficient* cause acts as cause when serving to complete a sufficient cause. The *etiogenetic fraction*/proportion for any given insufficient cause, conditional on cases of the illness having this cause as an antecedent, is the proportion of instances (person-moments) of the domain of the etiogenetic object of study such that the index history completes a sufficient cause but the reference history does not.

Note 5: A *necessary* cause of a given outcome is an insufficient cause that is a component in all minimally sufficient causes of that outcome.

Note 6: An agent that is definitional to a sickness or an illness is not a cause of it, much less a necessary cause. (See 'Agent' in sect. I – 1. 2.)

Superpopulation – In sampling theory, a hypothetical, abstract set of sampled units, infinite in size, the truth(s) about which is (are) the object(s) of inference.

Note: In statistical science the counterpart of superpopulation is the *domain* of the object of study.

Testability – See 'Quality of study object(s).'

Time – One of the two dimensions of the realm in which epidemiological phenomena take place, the other one being population, the two together constituting *population-time*. (Cf. space-time in modern, Einsteinian physics.)

Note 1: All (human) populations, whether closed (cohort-type) or open (dynamic), have their existence over time (longitudinally in time, i.e., diachronically); they are 'in motion' over time. A population's size integrated over a span of time (calendar time, say) amounts to an aggregate of population-time (measured in the units of person-years, say).

Note 2: Population-time is the realm in which *incidence density* takes manifestation.

Note 3: When members of a population are 'arrested' in their 'motions over time,' the result no longer is a population but, instead, a (stationary) *series of person-moments*. (This need not represent the population's 'cross-section' at a given time on a given scale of time, its members synchronously in this meaning.)

Note 4: A series of person-moments is the realm in which *proportion-type rates*, whether of incidence or prevalence, take manifestation.

Note 5: In a cohort's 'motion over time,' the time epidemiologically in question generally is *cohort time*, for the scale of which T_0 is the time of the membership-clinching event. A cohort's members enter the cohort simultaneously in cohort time, and they remain simultaneous in cohort time, for ever after. (See 'Cohort' in sect. II – 4.)

Note 6: In a dynamic population's 'motion over time,' epidemiologically in question generally is (Gregorian) *calendar time*, for the scale of which T_0 is not epidemiologically defined. (See 'Dynamic population' in sect. II – 4.)

Note 7: The phenomena (of occurrence) 'observed' in an epidemiological study have their temporal referents not only in cohort time (Note 5 above) or calendar time (Note 6 above) but always also in *study time*, for which T_0 is the time at which the process of data collection (possibly mere abstraction of data from a pre-existing database) begins.

Note 8: All of the data collection in an epidemiological study is *prospective* in study time (i.e., occurs in study time $T > T_0$), but the temporal referents of the data – some, or even all, of them – may be *retrospective* in study time. (The latter is particularly true of etiogenetic histories.)

Note 9: In an etiologic/etiogenetic study, the outcome events (of the illness occurring) take place at T_0 of *etiogenetic time*, and the etiogenetic histories are retrospective on this scale of *scientific time*. Thus, when the source and study populations are being followed over calendar time, the clock of scientific time shows $T = T_0$ at each point of calendar time; etiogenetic/scientific $T = T_0$ characterizes each person-moment in the study base.

Note 10: In an intervention study, the (or each) determinant contrast (between interventions) is formed as of T_0, and it is maintained prospectively (in $T > T_0$), in *intervention time*, in this genre of scientific time. The outcomes at issue occur in prospective scientific/intervention time, but determinants of the rate of any given outcome's occurrence may include ones that on this scale are retrospective (pre-T_0) in their temporal referents – these in addition to the prospective intervention. The study population being a cohort, the cohort time coincides (as for T_0, etc.) with the intervention/scientific time.

Note 11: Quite remarkably, *latency period** epidemiologic researchers (in occupational epidemiology in particular) commonly think of as "The interval between initiation of exposure to the causal agent and appearance or detection of the health process" [4]. This operational concept of latency period (cf. sect. I – 1. 2) would be admissible only if it could be presumed that the initiation of the exposure was an immediate, sufficient cause of the illness.

Note 12: As should be evident, it is *meaningless to characterize a study as either prospective or retrospective*; at issue can only be some particular aspect of (the object or methodology of) the study, on some particular scale of time. In particular, a study on the etiogenesis of a study is not prospective on the ground that its source-base is prospective in study time; nor is it retrospective on the ground that the determinant is retrospective in etiogenetic/scientific time. (A person is not healthy just because a particular organ system of his/hers is healthy.)

Trichotomous – Concerning an element in the object of study, the quality of being constituted by (only) three categories. (Cf. 'Dichotomous' and 'Polytomous.')

Note: A trichotomy is statistically represented by two indicator (0, 1) variates, indicating two of the three possible realizations.

*Variable** – "Any quantity that varies. Any attribute, phenomenon, or event that can have different values" [4].

Note: As this definition, like many others, indicates, among epidemiological researchers – and statisticians, too – it remains commonplace to fail to distinguish between characterizers of persons (the dimensions of age and gender, etc.) and statistical variables/variates (numerical) adopted (ad hoc) for representation of these (notably in regression models). But gender, for example, does not have "different values," only a gender variable/variate (statistical) does; nor does a health event have "different values," only an outcome variable/variate does; etc. (Cf. Note 2 under 'Exposure' and under 'Polytomous.')

II – 4. TERMS AND CONCEPTS OF METHODS OF STUDY

See note opening section II – 2.

*Accuracy** – See 'Accuracy and precision.'

Accuracy and precision – Concerning the result on – the empirical counterpart of – a parameter in statistical science (epidemiological, say), the respective referent concepts of 'accuracy' and 'precision' have become these (cf. sect. I – 2. 2):

Accuracy – The degree to which the empirical value accords with the theoretical one; that is, the degree to which an empirical magnitude, as a measure of a theoretical one, is free of error.

Precision (synonym: reproducibility) – The degree to which the empirical value of a parameter is reproducible in replications of the study.

Note 1: The error (inaccuracy) in a given result is the sum of two components: the particular degree of imprecision (chance error) in the result at issue (i.e., the ad hoc value of the random errors in the hypothetical replications) and the magnitude of *bias* in a study such as the one at issue (i.e., the typical error in the replications).

Note 2: The imprecision/irreproducibility of the result of a study (on a parameter's magnitude) has two sources: the limited *size* of the study and the wanting *efficiency* of it. Even with the maximal possible efficiency, infinite size would generally be needed for complete freedom from imprecision.

*Adjustment** – In a causal (generally etiogenetic) study, replacement of the crude result (generally for RR) by its counterpart conditional on (some) confounders. (See 'Control of confounding.')

Admissibility (synonym: eligibility) – Concerning a person or person-moment, the quality of meeting all of the criteria necessary for admission into the study base; also: concerning the study methodology at large, its consistency with the imperatives of ethics (cf. 'Institutional Review Board' in sect. III – 4).

Note 1: A person's admissibility – eligibility for admission – into a study does not mean that admission should result.

Note 2: In the context of a scientific study, the criteria of admissibility are, generally, scientific in part only; the rest of them have to do with practicalities of the study. Examples of the latter: area of residence, language, and being compos mentis.

O. S. Miettinen, *Epidemiological Research: Terms and Concepts*,
DOI 10.1007/978-94-007-1171-6_7, © Springer Science+Business Media B.V. 2011

Age group – A (common) misnomer for an age category, for a range of age. (Cf. 'Category.')

Analysis of data – See 'Data analysis.'

Ancillary study – A study exploiting the database of a study conducted for some other purpose.

*Association** – See sect. II – 3.

Note 1: Like any result of an empirical study, the association documented in a study to test an etiogenetic hypothesis is *descriptive* of experience; but it is *intended* to reflect causality – with confounder-adjustment commonly the means to this end.

Note 2: Once the hypothesis has become reasonably well-established as a piece of knowledge, attention turns to the corresponding occurrence relation in terms of a regression function which accounts for the causal rate-ratio's dependence on its modifiers. (Cf. Note 5 under 'Causal rate-ratio' in sect. II – 3.)

Assumption – The term is a (common) misnomer for the presumption (of correctness) represented by the statistical model being deployed. (Cf. sect. I – 2. 2, 3. 2.)

Note: Presumption is the statistical-science counterpart of assumption in statistics.

*Attributable risk** – See 'Attributable and relative risk.'

*Attributable and relative risk** – Traditional terms for two central concepts in epidemiology, only gradually being replaced by the corresponding apposite ones: 'rate difference' and 'rate ratio,' respectively [5]. (See 'Risk' in sect. I – 1. 2.)

Note: These terms are particularly inappropriate for the difference and ratio, respectively, of *empirical* rates (risk being a singularly theoretical concept).

Base – See 'Study base.'

*Baseline** – Concerning follow-up, the (point in) time at which it begins.

Note: At issue generally is follow-up of (members of) a cohort, and baseline in this naturally is the zero-point of cohort time.

*Base population** (synonym: study population) – See 'Study population.'

*Bias** – Consequence of study methodology such that even with infinite study size the result (free of imprecision) would be at variance with the parameter value at issue; also: the extent of this discrepancy.

Note 1: In *hypothesis-testing* about the etiogenesis of an illness, *descriptive* validity requires, for one, that the median of the result's replication-distribution be $RR = 1$ conditionally on the absence of the association (theoretical) at issue; and for another, that it be in the RR > 1 range conditionally on the association – whatever value (however quantitatively invalid) in the RR > 1 range.

Note 2: In a study for *quantification* of etiogenetic effect, *descriptive* validity requires that the median of the result's (empirical RR's) replication distribution accord with the corresponding theoretical value (descriptive, conditional on the specifics in the designed object for the quantification study) conditionally on whatever theoretical value of the RR (non-null as well as null).

Note 3: Incompleteness of descriptive validity in etiogenetic studies is of two broad types: *selection* bias and *documentation* bias.

Note 4: Insofar as the result of an etiogenetic study is taken to be a measure not merely of an association (descriptive) but of the *causal* relation of etiogenetic interest, validity involves the added requirement of freedom (complete) from *confounding*, from confounding bias.

Note 5: Validity of a hypothesis-testing study on etiogenesis is consistent with biased documentation so long as the consequence of this is merely 'dilution' of the extent to which the empirical RR tends to exceed unity when the association (theoretical) does obtain.

Note 6: In derivative research, an important form of selection bias is *publication* bias. It results from result-dependent publication of original studies. (A system of studies' preregistration would prevent publication bias in derivative studies focused on registered studies irrespective of their publication.)

Biased base – In an original study, study base chosen with a hunch as to what the result from it, specifically, will be, or regarding which there should have been such a hunch; and in a derivative study, even in the context of original studies each with an unbiased base, the inclusion of original studies in a result-dependent way (cf. 'Publication bias' in Note 6 under 'Bias.')

Note 1: In valid research one 'consults' ad-hoc facts without any hunch as to what those particular facts were or will be.

Note 2: Biased choice of the base for a study is tantamount to *selection bias* in the study. Much confusion surrounds the meaning of 'selection bias,' as is manifest in the I.E.A. dictionary [4], most notably.

Note 3: In an etiogenetic study, the base is biased if the case series (and thereby the study base) is retrospective in study time and is formed because of a sense that a particular antecedent, potentially etiogenetic, seems to be notably common among the patients with the illness.

Biased documentation – Documentation of the pattern of occurrence in the study base in such a way that the study result is at variance with this pattern, specifically when the result deviates in a knowable direction from what the pattern (descriptive) actually was.

Note 1: As causation is not a phenomenon (but, instead, a noumenon), errors of documentation can only be errors of *description* of the phenomenal pattern, even in causal research. (Cf. 'Result.')

Note 2: Incomplete *detection of cases* of the outcome does not conduce to biased documentation (of rate ratio) in an etiogenetic study so long as the probability of detection (given the outcome) is independent of the etiogenetic history at issue. Yet, history-dependent detection of the outcome – due to history-dependent seeking of care and/or diagnosis (rule-in) is an important source of documentation bias in etiogenetic research, notably when the etiogenetic connection already is known (or strongly suspected). (This bias can be preventable by focus on cases that are severe and typical at that.)

Note 3: Apart from history-dependent case-detection, an equally eminent potential source of documentation bias in etiogenetic studies is outcome-dependent *history-documentation.*

Note 4: A notable third source of documentation bias in etiogenetic studies is biased *sampling* of the study base (for the base series).

Note 5: Misclassification of etiogenetic histories, so long as it is non-differential between the case and base series, is not a source of documentation bias in etiogenetic hypothesis-testing (cf. Notes 1 and 5 under 'Bias').

Biased result – The result from a (methodologically) biased study; also: the result from (the application of) a biased method of measurement (of a magnitude).

Note: The result of an epidemiological study can be thought of as the result of measurement directed to some parameter(s) of Nature, for assessment of the magnitude of this/these. This is so even in hypothesis-testing about an effect, even though the result is used merely in an effort to discriminate between null and non-null magnitudes of the comparative parameter.

Biased sampling – In sampling of the study base (for the base/referent series) in an etiogenetic/etiognostic or intervention-prognostic study [9], the use of an invalid method.

Note 1: The method of sampling for the base series is invalid if conditionally on the determinants in the occurrence relation being studied, including the matching factors, the sampling is not valid about the relative frequencies of the histories in the causal contrast at issue (specifically these conditional frequencies in the study base).

Note 2: Biasedness of the base series as a series per se is a topic distinct from that of the documented information on (the person-moments constituting) the series.

Note 3: Biased sampling for the base series is a potential element in the *documentation bias* of a study (distinct from selection and confounding biases; cf. Notes 3 and 5 under 'Bias').

Biased selection – See 'Biased base' (Note 2) and 'Biased sampling.'

Biased study – A study with selection and/or documentation bias descriptively, and/or confounding bias if the result is taken to be about an effect. (Cf. 'Bias.')

*Case** – A common misnomer for a person with a case of a particular illness (especially in the context of 'case-control' studies). (Cf. sect. I – 1. 2.)

*Case-base study** (synonym: case-referent study) – An eminent descriptive (rather than definitional) feature of the (structure of) the etiologic/etiogenetic study. (See 'Etiologic study.')

*Case-control study** (synonyms: retrospective study, case-history study) – "The observational epidemiological study of persons with the disease (or other outcome variable) of interest and a suitable control group of persons without the disease (comparison group, reference group). The potential relationship of a suspected risk factor or an attribute to the disease is examined by comparing the diseased and nondiseased with regard to how frequently the attribute or factor is present ... in each of the groups (diseased and nondiseased) [refs.]" [4].

Note 1: Instead of the persons involved, studied is an occurrence relation (abstract).

Note 2: Even though the term 'case-control study' is commonly – including in the I.E.A. dictionary [4] – used as a synonym for 'case-base study' and 'case-referent study,' the concept of 'case-control study' actually is profoundly different from the referent of those two other terms.

Note 3: The concept of 'case-control' study – or 'trohoc' (heteropalindrome of 'cohort') study – is seriously malformed. It represents what may be termed the *trohoc fallacy* (corresponding to the cohort fallacy). A case series (not group) in any epidemiological study has its meaning only in the context of its referent, the study base, in reference to which it presumably is the totality of cases. Its associated non-case series (not group), in turn, has meaning only if it is a fair sample of the person-moments (infinite in number) constituting the population-time of the study base. And once the two series are thus construed, comparison between them – numerator and denominator series – is seen to be profoundly misguided. Very notably, the alternative to causality – confounding, that is – can never be understood in terms of the "case-control" comparison – but only in terms of the etiogenetic contrast in reference to the study base. (See 'Directionality,' 'Overmatching,' and 'Etiologic study.')

Note 4: The terms 'retrospective study' and 'case-history study' have lost favor in comparison with 'case-control study,' while the respective concepts – fundamental fallacies – are the very same. (Cf. 'Etiologic study.')

*Case-referent study** (synonym: case-base study) – See 'Case-base study' and 'Etiologic study.'

*Case series** – A set of instances, notably of an illness (or sickness or death).

Catchment population – See 'Source population' (Note 2).

Causal contrast – Contrast of two experiences, one with the cause (potential) present and the other with its alternative present, as to the respective rates (or other measures) of the outcome's occurrence with a view to causal inference (inductive) based on the pattern. (Cf. sect. II – 3.)

Note: Such a contrast produces an empirical value for a *comparative parameter* – in an etiogenetic study for a rate ratio, supposed to be conditional on all material confounders of the study base. This value is *descriptive* of the experience; and however valid it may be as a measure of the phenomenal association in the study base, it is but an input to the inference about the effect – unobservable, noumenal.

Causal criteria/considerations* – "Considerations (often called 'criteria') that help to guide judgments about causality and to make causal inferences [refs.]. Examples close to epidemiology include John Stuart Mill's canons, the 'rules' of David Hume, Evan's postulates, Henle-Koch postulates, or [*sic*] Hill's criteria [*sic*] of causation" [4].

Note 1: Most recognizable – famous – in medicine at large are those Henle-Koch 'postulates.' But from the vantage of etiologic/etiogenetic research they are of no consequence. For, they actually pertain to making an agent definitional, rather than causal, to an illness, as in tuberculosis, silicosis, etc. [23].

Note 2: In modern epidemiology, most eminent by far are *A. B. Hill*'s answers [41] to his question about "an association between two variables, perfectly clear-cut and beyond what we would care to attribute to the play of chance." His question was, "What aspects of that association should we especially consider before deciding that the most likely interpretation is causation?" The answers he formulated with special reference to *occupational etiogenesis* of illness:

"*Strength.* First upon my list I would put the strength of the association. . . .

"*Consistency.* Next on my list of features to be specially considered I would place the consistency of the observed association. Has it been repeatedly observed by different persons, in different places, circumstances, and times? . . .

"*Specificity.* [This quality] of the association [is] the third characteristic which invariably we must consider. If . . . the association is limited to specific workers and to particular sites and types of disease and there is no association between the work and other modes of dying, then clearly that is a strong argument in favor of causation.

"*Temporality.* My fourth characteristic is the temporal relationship of the association . . . which might be particularly relevant with diseases of slow development. . . .

"*Biological gradient.* Fifthly, if the association is one which can reveal a biological gradient, or dose-response curve, then we should look most carefully for such evidence. . . .

"*Plausibility.* It will be helpful if the causation we suspect is biologically plausible. . . .

"*Coherence.* On the other hand the cause-and-effect interpretation of our data should not seriously conflict with the generally known facts of the natural history and biology of the disease. . . .

"*Experiment.* Occasionally it is possible to appeal to experimental, or semi-experimental, evidence. . . .

"*Analogy*. In some circumstances it would be fair to judge by analogy. . . ."

Note 3: These Hill 'considerations' are of great eminence in the annals of epidemiological research, in part because Hill worked very extensively with R. Doll, most famously on smoking etiogenesis of lung cancer; and the article at issue here appeared soon after the landmark *Smoking and Health* report of the U. S. Surgeon General (in 1964). Viewed from the vantage of the present, very notable is the non-inclusion, among these 'considerations,' of the topic of *confounding*.

Note 4: Now, almost half-a-century on, a substantially *different conceptual framework* for causal inference in etiogenetic research is a consideration:

1. Members of the relevant *scientific community* have their respective, subjective *prior* probabilities of the correctness of the hypothesis, based on considerations other than the epidemiological evidence.

2. Members of the relevant scientific community, concerned to update their non-epidemiological priors on the basis of epidemiological evidence, need to appreciate this *overarching canon* for viewing the evidence: If the occurrence of an outcome is (positively) associated with an antecedent conditionally on all potential *confounders*, then the antecedent is etiogenetic to the outcome. (In this, the antecedent – in principle potentially causal – is viewed in terms of the duality inherent in the hypothesis: antecedent present vs. its alternative present; index category vs. reference category of the potential risk factor.) And they also need to appreciate that it generally is *very challenging* to get to a justifiable belief about whether this association (descriptive) actually obtains (in the abstract).

3. In an *ideal* world for etiogenetic inference, the entirety of the epidemiological evidence would be in secure conformity with that overarching canon, securely known to be *fully free from bias* – not only from selection and documentation bias but from residual confounding bias also – and, thus, limited only in its precision/informativeness. Available would be, on this basis, the likelihood function from the ideal and ultimately solely relevant derivative study. Using this LF together with their respective prior probabilities for the correctness of the hypothesis, members of the relevant scientific community would derive, in the way of Bayesian statistics, their respective *posterior* probabilities – as inputs for consensus-seeking in the relevant scientific community (select representatives of this).

4. In the *real* world, such as it actually is, an essential, very challenging preparatory phase before the inference is *adjustment* – as a subjective, judgmental surmise – of the result from each original study for the biases in it. These then need to be translated into their joint implication for the derivative result; and the latter, in turn, needs to be adjusted for the publication bias in it. Realistically, Bayesian formalism scarcely has a role in this.

5. From the vantage of this outlook, the Hill 'considerations' can be given their respective meanings:

Strength. The idea that causal associations tend to be "strong" (causal RR >> 1) – insofar as this indeed is someone's belief – means that the values of RR in the non-null range (of RR > 1) close to RR = 1 are given relatively low *prior* probabilities (i.e., that the cumulative prior is rather flat in this near-null range, following the 'jump' at RR = 1).

Consistency. In respect to this "consideration," Hill lost consistency of his train of thought and presentation: even though at issue was going to be causal interpretation of an association that is "perfectly clear-cut and beyond what we would care to attribute to chance," under "consistency" he said that "whether chance is the explanation or whether a true hazard has been revealed may sometimes be answered only by a repetition of the circumstances and the observations"; and it is not "sometimes" but usually that replication of a first study is called for. The dream of consistent results in replications actually has to do with the same domain of the object of study, with no significance to "different persons in different places, at different times." Replication is not a matter of seeking diversity in terms of "quite a wide variety of situations and techniques" (as in the research on smoking etiogenesis of illness) – with the idea of putting "a good deal of weight upon similar results reached in quite different ways, e.g., prospectively and retrospectively," thinking that on this basis "we can justifiably infer that the association is not due to some consistent error or fallacy that permeates every inquiry." The idea in replications is not that of seeking to reproduce previous results with the original errors and/or fallacies but without them, if any are identified. Hill drew rather heavily on the "lesson" of the studies on smoking etiogenesis of lung cancer but did not mention the discovery having been made – and translated into public policies – in Nazi Germany already [42].

Specificity. Under "Specificity" Hill returned to causal interpretation of an association the existence (abstract) of which is not in question. He noted, with understanding, that "the prospective investigations of smoking and cancer of the lung have been criticized for not showing specificity – in other words the death rate of smokers is higher than the death rate of non-smokers from many causes of death ..." This is to say that, for example, the *prior* probability (subjective) of smoking being etiogenetic to coronary heart disease generally is, or at least should be, reduced by the knowledge that smoking is etiogenetic to lung cancer. Today's epidemiologists scarcely agree with this, as they think of, say, obesity and sedentary life-style as being etiogenetic for a large variety of illnesses.

Temporality. For any hypothesis that something subsequent to the occurrence of an illness is etiogenetic to it, the *prior* probability generally is, and always should be, zero.

Biological gradient. Hill wrote that "the fact that the death rate from cancer of the lung rises linearly with the number of cigarettes smoked daily, adds a very great deal to the simpler evidence that cigarette smokers have a higher death rate than non-smokers." But today, now that we have the idea of confoundedness being the alternative to causality of an outcome-antecedent association, it is possible and necessary to appreciate that confounded associations, too, are prone to show 'dose-response.' For example, the yellower has been the index finger, the higher is the risk of lung cancer.

Plausibility. At issue in this is, naturally, the *prior* probability of the association's causality, uninfluenced by the epidemiological evidence.

Coherence. Having remarked on the inferential relevance of coherence of the association in epidemiological studies with, for example, the population-level temporal correspondence between mortality from lung cancer and consumption of cigarettes, Hill digressed again: "Personally, I regard as greatly contributing to coherence the histopathological evidence from the bronchial epithelium of smokers and the isolation from cigarette smoke of factors carcinogenic to the skin of laboratory animals," adding that "such laboratory evidence can enormously strengthen the hypothesis . . ." This has to do with extra-epidemiological influences on the plausibility of the causal hypothesis, *prior* to the epidemiological evidence, even though "coherence," like "strength," for example, was set forth as one of the "aspects of that association [we should] especially consider before deciding that the most likely interpretation of it is causation." (As for coherence of the epidemiological evidence, Doll was puzzled by negative association, among smokers, between inhalation of the smoke and risk of lung cancer.)

Experiment. Hill actually did not refer to experiments but to *negative* association of the illness with *reduction* in the potentially causal antecedent: "The dust in the workshop is reduced, lubricating oils are changed, persons stop smoking cigarettes. Is the frequency of the associated events changed? Here the strongest support for the causation hypothesis may be revealed." But it is inapparent why negative association of lung cancer with quitting smoking should be viewed as more strongly suggestive of causation than positive association with taking up smoking. Of course, genuinely experimental evidence would be more compelling than any non-experimental association if there were genuine (rather than R. A. Fisher's industry-sponsored) concern about possible but undocumentable confoundedness of the latter.

Analogy. "With the effects of thalidomide and rubella before us we would surely be ready to accept slighter but similar evidence with another drug or another viral disease in pregnancy," Hill wrote. But again, the topic is not an aspect of the association at issue but influences on epidemiologists' *prior* probabilities concerning the existence of the hypothesized etiogenesis.

*Causal inference** – In the context of evidence from an epidemiological study (original or derivative), use of this evidence to inductively 'update' one's view (subjective) about the existence or the magnitude of the effect (in the domain at issue). (See also 'Causal criteria/considerations.')

Note 1: The point of departure in causal inference is one's *prior-probability function*, expressing one's probability that the effect-measure's magnitude (M) is smaller than a particular value (m) for various – indeed all – possible values of the latter; that is, $\Pr(M < m)$ as a (cumulative) function of m. The inference, then, is the translation of this function into its corresponding *posterior-probability function*, as one sees to be warranted in the face of the evidence. At issue is the effect-measure's magnitude in the abstract.

Note 2: Implied by Note 1 above is that even in the non-null situation the effect-measure has a singular magnitude; but this is, quite generally, unrealistic. Therefore, both of those probability functions in respect to the non-null range(s) need to be taken to refer to the study domain with modifier-distributions such as they were in the experience(s) addressed by the evidence. Of course, inference about the non-null magnitudes in these aggregative terms is of little consequence, as it is the modifier-conditional magnitudes that really matter for practice. But, if the causal connection is thus inferred to exist, the mind is open to the quantitative particulars from suitably valid empirical regression functions.

Note 3: Apart from having to contend with the quantitative implications of the modifier-distribution in the evidentiary experience(s) in reference to the non-null situation (Note 2 above), the inferential statistic – the *likelihood function* – from the evidence poses very considerable, if not insurmountable, challenges in addition. For, it quite commonly needs adjustments before it is valid for *causal* inference (à la Note 1 above), and very difficult judgments (subjective) are needed for these. The substantive/causal null state (of no effect) does not inherently coincide with the statistical/descriptive null state of no association (with such conditionality of it as characterizes the evidence), and the LF thus needs to be adjusted for the presumed biases in the results, including the degree of residual confounding in each of the results at hand. And the derivative result generally needs adjustment for publication bias besides. (Cf. Note 4 under 'Causal criteria/considerations.')

Note 4: In these terms, inference based on the result of a study (original or derivative) pertaining to the correctness/incorrectness of a causal hypothesis (yes, the hypothesis, rather than its denial) is development – very challenging, judgemental – of the change in the probability (subjective) of the correctness of its denial; that is, update of the null state's prior probability to its posterior probability. And as for the magnitude of the effect-measure (aggregative, à la Note 2 above), a *point estimate* is the median of someone's posterior-probability function, and the corresponding $100(1 - \alpha)\%$ *interval estimate* is the parameter's range from 2.5% to 97.5% in the (cumulative) posterior-probability function.

Note 5: As is thus evident, inference about an effect (etiogenetic, say) is not something the result of which can be read from the numerical evidence, from the 'inferential' statistic(s); it is a mental process that involves subjective probability and judgment, and the end result of it has a strong subjective element (in addition to the evidence) behind it. It follows that, for the purposes of etiogenetic epidemiological research, *frequentist inference* is a contradiction-in-terms, and that its 'point estimate' (mere empirical value) and 'confidence interval' (mere P-value difference interval) are seriously misleading misnomers. Moreover, while *Bayesian inference* has a theoretically tenable framework for inductive inference in the context of objectively valid evidence, in non-experimental etiogenetic research the RR result is not an objectively valid measure (empirical) of the effect at issue. (Cf. 'Estimate' in sect. I – 3. 2 and Note 4 under 'Causal criteria/considerations.')

Cause-probability score – See 'Propensity score.'

Centile* (synonym: percentile) – Concerning a distribution on a *continuous* scale, the point on that scale such that a given percentage of the distribution falls to the left of it. (Examples: 95th centile is the value at which the cumulative probability is 0.95 or 95%; the 50th centile is the median.) Concerning a *discrete* distribution, a given centile, thus defined, may not exist at all; but if it does, it generally has a range, as cumulative probability is flat between its 'jumps' at the discrete realizations. (Example: For a Bernoulli distribution with $P < 0.80$ there is no quintile; the cumulative probability is $1 - P > 0.20$ for all values in the 0-to-1 range except for the 'jump' to this value at realization 0, and from this to 1 at realization 1.) (Cf. 'Distribution function.')

Note: Different from 'percentile,' 'centile' as a word rhymes with the words for other *fractiles*. (See 'Fractile.')

CI – Confidence interval.

*Closed population**** (synonym: cohort) – See 'Cohort' (Note 1).

*Coding**** – See 'Data.'
Note: Failure to distinguish between data-coding and variate-definition (for 'data analysis') remains commonplace. In common epidemiological parlance (and writings, too), age and gender, for example, are 'variables' (rather than characterizers of persons). The distinction matters, because the coding does not, inherently, define the variate or variates that are to be based on it. For example, if age is coded in terms of the number of years, there commonly is a need to derive more than one variate from this (for the linear compound in a regression model); and there are various possible ways of doing this.

*Cohort**** (synonym: closed population) – A population whose membership is defined by (the occurrence of) a particular event (in the context of certain prerequisites, perhaps), lasting forever thereafter [12]. (Example: For the cohort in the Framingham Heart Study, the membership-defining event was the enrolment, one of the prerequisites for this being residency in Framingham. No-one entering this population has lost membership in it, not by loss-to-follow-up nor by intentional termination of follow-up – nor, for that matter, by death.) (Cf. 'Dynamic population.')
Note 1: A cohort is a *closed* population in the meaning of being closed for exit: once a member, always a member. (Gr. *cohors*, 'enclosure.')
Note 2: While the term 'cohort' has been well-established among epidemiological researchers, its meaning has not been. The teaching has been that, in ancient Rome, *cohors* meant (presumably among its other meanings) one of the 10 divisions of a legion (of soldiers); and that once a cohort (in this meaning) had been recruited, new members were not recruited in replacement of those who died. This idea is now surviving under the term and concept of "fixed cohort" – a cohort "in which no additional membership is allowed" [4].
Note 3: Failure to understand the conceptually crisp duality constituted by cohort-type, closed populations and dynamic, open populations [12] – 'dynamic' referring to turnover of membership – has recently led to the strikingly malformed

term and concept of "dynamic cohort": "a population that gains and loses members," where "cohort" means "any designated group of persons who are followed or traced over a period of time" [4].

Note 4: A population is whatever it is irrespective of whether it is "designated" for something or is "followed or traced over a period of time." And insofar as "group" (Note 3) is meant to refer to a type of population (which inherently exists over time), it must mean a cohort rather than a dynamic population (such as the resident population of Framingham, from which the FHS cohort was recruited). (Cf. 'Group.')

Cohort fallacy – See 'Cohort study' (Notes 3 and 4).

Cohort study* (synonyms: prospective study, follow-up study) – A study addressing etiology/etiogenesis, one in which "subsets of a defined population can be identified who are, have been, or in the future may be exposed or not exposed, or exposed in different degrees, to a factor or factors hypothesized to influence the occurrence of a disease or other outcome [refs.]. The main feature of a cohort study is observation of large numbers over a long period (commonly years), with comparison of incidence rates in groups that differ in exposure levels" [4].

Note 1: The Framingham Heart Study has been held as the paradigmatic cohort study. But it – like the subsequent, equally famous Nurses' Health Study (at Harvard) – was originally designed as a program of prospective *data-collection*, on the recruited cohort, for the purposes of a *multitude of studies*, unspecified at the time of the cohort's formation (in 1948-1949). Neither the FHS nor the NHS has been *a* (single) study. Nor, by the way, is the NHS about the health of nurses; in it, experience with nurses is (documented and) used to learn about women's health.

Note 2: The concept of cohort study as a type of etiogenetic study actually has been this: A cohort is enrolled as the study population. In it, the etiogenetic histories are ascertained, once and for all, at the time of enrolment (at cohort T_0). The cohort is followed for documentation of the outcome event of interest. And then, the prospective occurrence of the outcome is related to the retrospective divergence of the etiogenetic determinant (defined at cohort T_0).

Note 3: This conception of an etiogenetic study (Note 2 above) – actually of the ideal study in this genre (given its generally inescapable non-experimental nature) – arose as an emulation of the randomized trial in intervention-prognostic research; but the result of adopting this false paradigm got to be the *cohort fallacy*. In a randomized trial, quite rationally, prospective occurrence – in a cohort – is addressed in relation to prospective divergence in the causal determinant, while in a 'cohort study' (etiogenetic), rather irrationally, prospective occurrence is addressed in relation to retrospective divergence in the causal determinant (Note 2 above). (In this, 'prospective' and 'retrospective' refer to cohort time, the zero point of which is the time of enrolment, the same for each member of the cohort, even though the enrolments differ in their respective points in calendar time; cf. Note 5 under 'Time' in sect. II – 3.)

Note 4: In any recovery from the cohort fallacy, the beginning is the realization that the cohort in a so-called cohort study actually is but the *source population* for the study, and that the cohort's follow-up actually defines the *source base* of the study. With this much understood, the 'cohort study' naturally gets to be transformed into *the* etiologic study, just as liberation from the trohoc fallacy, constituted by the 'case-control study,' leads to *the* etiologic study (cf. 'Etiologic study.')

Note 5: Insofar as the term 'cohort study' is to be retained in the lexicons of epidemiology, two things should be understood: first, that its (logical) alternative is 'dynamic-population study'; and second, that the corresponding conceptual duality (in types of source population) is quite trivial, the study population being dynamic regardless.

Cohort time – See 'Time' (Notes 5 and 10) in section II – 3.

*Community trial** – An experimental intervention-prognostic study for community medicine (as distinct from clinical trial, for clinical medicine).

Note 1: An inherent feature of a community trial is that the units of (allocation and) observation are populations (as distinct from individuals in clinical trials) [4].

Note 2: Remarkably, even though epidemiologists view screening for a cancer as inherently being a matter of community-level preventive medicine (which it isn't), they insist on *clinical* trials in the assessment of the reduction in (community-level) mortality from the cancer, resulting from the screening's introduction into a community – and great confusion is the result of the confusion, both ontic and epistemic, in this research [33, 43, 44].

Comparability – Concerning the compared subpopulations within a study population, their suitability for the comparison at issue.

Note 1: In an etiologic/etiogenetic study, comparability of the index and reference segments of the study base requires that the causal histories represent a *meaningfully construed causal contrast* (sect. II – 3).

Note 2: The operationalized causal contrast must represent comparability in terms of *extraneous aspects of the compared categories*, about freedom from confounding by these. Example: If, in a study of the etiogenesis of lung cancer, at issue is an air-borne agent and the index history – the agent's presence – is represented by work in one of a particular set of work-sites and the reference history – the agent's absence – by work in another particular set of work-sites, the contrasted sites need to be similar in terms of other types of air-borne carcinogens.

Note 3: Comparability in an etiogenetic study does not require similarity of the *compared populations* in respect to their distributions by such well-documentable extraneous determinants of the outcome's occurrence – such potential confounders – as age and gender, as their control (so as to assure unconfounded result) is feasible. Socio-economic status, if relevant (as in etiogenetic studies having to do with lung cancer), poses a considerable problem of comparability, to be solved by prevention (in the formation of the study base) rather than by documentation-and-control.

Note 4: Comparability also has to do with the identification and documentation of – that is, with the information about – the outcome's occurrences. Comparability generally requires that the *case identification* be independent of the causal history, specifically for the cases as they are defined for inclusion in the case series (notably as to how typical and how severe).

*Comparison group/population** (synonym: reference group/population) – A group/population representing a determinant category or domain different from that of express interest, used to put the experience with the former in a meaning-enhancing perspective. (Cf. 'Control group.')

Conclusion – Based on a study, a firm inference – inductive – about the abstract truth that was the object of the study. (Cf. sect. I – 2. 2.)

Note: Conclusions from epidemiological research studies (scientific) are, as a rule, *unjustifiable*. Yet, editors of epidemiologic and other medical journals demand conclusion to be presented, not in the body of each study report but, incongruously with this, in the report's Abstract or Summary. This practice is indefensible and should be discontinued. (Cf. 'Study' in sect. I – 2. 2 and 'Causal inference' above.)

*Confidence interval** – See 'Estimate' in section 1 – 3. 2 and 'Causal inference' (Note 5).

Note: This is a misnomer for what actually is the study result's *imprecision* interval.

Confounder adjustment – See 'Control of confounding.'

Confounder score – See 'Control of confounding' (Notes 2-5).

*Confounding** – In an outcome's empirical association with an antecedent – descriptively valid association, possibly nil in magnitude ($RR = 1$), with an antecedent that in principle could be causal (see Note 1 below) – the possible explanation, partial or full, other than the antecedent's degree of role (when present) in the outcome's etiology/etiogenesis.

Note 1: For possibly being a cause, an antecedent must allow for a *causal contrast* with its alternative in each instance from the study domain (sect. II – 3). This is not the case, most notably, with a person's age and gender (in the traditional meaning of the gender chromosome complement, XX or XY). A given person having been born at a (substantially) different time or with the other gender was not a possible alternative for what got to be, with the person remaining (what we think of as) the same person.

Note 2: At issue in respect to potential confounding is an outcome-antecedent association that is either the crude association (in terms of RR) or one conditional on certain confounders; and it issue are, respectively, the full (amount of) confounding prior to its control and the residual confounding after its control. A descriptively valid association fully *conditional* on all confounders would be a purely causal association. (Such an association presumably is extremely rare in epidemiological research.)

Note 3: Confounding as an explanation (partial at least) of a descriptively valid possibly-causal association has to do with confounders in the meaning of *extraneous determinants* of the outcome's occurrence, imbalanced in their distributions between the index (cause present) and reference (the alternative present) segments of the study base. Specifically, confounders are determinants (extraneous) of the outcome's occurrence conditionally on the causal determinant's *reference category* (in which the implications of effect-modification are not an issue).

Note 4: Confounders *need not be causal* determinants of the outcome's occurrence – as exemplified by (the common role of) age and gender as confounders (cf. Note 1 above).

Note 5: *Control* of confounding – by replacing the crude association by one that is conditional on the confounder(s) – is to be distinguished from *prevention* of confounding – by making the index and reference segments of the study base have (essentially) identical distributions by (some of the recognized potential) confounders.

Note 6: In judgments about the residual confounding in an association produced by an etiologic/etiogenetic study, say, an important qualitative distinction is that between *positive* and *negative* confounding; that is, between confounding that adds to the magnitude of the association and confounding that takes away from it (possibly even turning an otherwise positive association into a negative one).

Note 7: In etiologic/etiogenetic research, confounding – notably residual confounding – is typically positive in the direction of its consequence. For, causes of illness tend to be positively correlated within the principal genera of these: a constitutional cause tends to be positively correlated with other constitutional ones; analogously for behavioral and environmental hazards to health.

*Confounding bias** – See 'Bias' (Note 4) and 'Confounding.'

*Control** – The act of forming an artificial setting – study base – in which the empirical counterpart of the object of study (an occurrence relation) was or will be documented (as opposed to merely selecting/assembling the study base from what is 'naturally' available); that is, the act(s) definitional to an experiment (its 'controlled' setting); also: removal of confounding from study result, when the study base and, hence, the crude result are confounded; and also: a member of the 'control group' in a 'case-control study.'

Note: Experimental control is not a feature of only causality-oriented studies; it can be a feature of a descriptive study. Example: In a study intended to serve improvement of case-finding among contacts of a person with a communicable disease, the artificial introduction, ad hoc, of a 'naturally' still non-existing diagnostic test suitable for application by an epidemiologist in 'field' conditions.

*Control group** (synonym: reference group) – In an intervention study, the group (subcohort) serving to provide information about an important counterfactual concerning the intervention/index group (subcohort): that which would have been the course of health in this group, had the intervention had no effect.

Note 1: The control/reference group in an intervention study is from the same domain as the intervention/index group, different from any comparison group in relation to the group of interest in a descriptive study. (Cf. 'Comparison group.')

Note 2: The term is a misnomer for a misconstrued element in the trohoc fallacy. (See Note 3 under 'Case-control study.')

Note 3: The control group needs to satisfy comparability with the index group even though it is not there for comparison.

Control of confounding* – In the context of documented confounding of the study base, seeing to it that this does not translate into confoundedness of the study result.

Note 1: The *means* of controlling confounding are, broadly, these: (1) mutual standardization of the compared rates (as entries into the comparative measure, standardized rate-ratio, say); (2) formulating the comparative measure within strata based on the confounder(s) and deriving the overall measure from these (by, e.g., the M-H principle); and (3) making adjustment(s) for the confounding in the framework of (multiple) regression 'analysis.' A combination of #2 and #3 involves stratification by a regression-based confounder score [45].

Note 2: Confounder-adjustment by means of regression 'analysis' has the drawback of lack of transparency – the need of the study report's readers to take the attained confounder-conditionality on faith. The solution to this problem is the development of a regression-based confounder score for each of the person-moments in the study series – the case and base series (see 'Etiologic study') – and the formation of strata on the basis of these score-values (as though stratifying by age alone). The confounders can be shown to have balanced distributions between the index and reference person-moments within the strata, thus making plain the attainment of conditionality on the confounders [45].

Note 3: In the context of several confounders to be controlled – adjusted for – approaches 1 and 2 in Note 1 above are impractical on the ground of major loss of information (about the RR). It is to this problem that regression 'analysis' is the first-order solution; and to its opaqueness, stratification by the unidimensional confounder-score – with no cross-stratification needed – is the solution [45].

Note 4: Given that confounders are characterized by their associations with both the outcome and the determinant at issue, the multivariate scoring function for use in stratification can in principle address the occurrence (in the study base) of the outcome or, alternatively, of the (potential) cause at issue [45]. Two considerations generally favor the use of scoring having to do with the propensity for the outcome's occurrence: this, different from the cause's occurrence, is of scientific interest; and the outcome's occurrence routinely translates into the realization of a (scalar-valued) simple variate – Bernoulli-distributed (in the two series forming the database), providing for logistic regression – whereas the determinant histories tend to be represented by more than one variate.

Note 5: When holding the randomized trial as the paradigm for the etiologic study – unjustifiable though this is [9] – the concern is to form strata within which the propensities to fall in the causal determinant's contrasted categories are the same (as though randomly assigned); and from this vantage the preference naturally is for determinant-oriented propensity-scoring.

Note 6: A necessary concomitant of control of confounding is that the precision of the confounder-conditional measure of association is addressed with the same conditioning – as when combining the M-H 'point estimate' and the M-H test statistic's realization in deriving a 'test-based interval estimate' [46].

*Cost** – See 'Efficiency' (Note 1).

*Cross-validation** – See 'Validation' (Note).

*Data** – The aggregate of information collected and documented in a study.

Note: The data undergo transformations. In the first phase collected and documented are *primary* data (as in filling out a questionnaire). These are translated into *coded* data, for storage and retrieval (using a computer). And these, in turn, are translated into realizations of the statistical variates in the object of study, into *statistical* data in this meaning.

Data analysis – The process of deriving one or more *statistics* from the database produced by a study. Specifically, given the data in the form of realizations for the statistical variates in the designed (form of the) occurrence relation that is the object of study or definitional to the object of study, translation of the corresponding (matrix of) statistical data into the corresponding statistics (e.g., into the parameters' empirical/fitted values and the SEs of these, by fitting the occurrence relation's logistic counterpart to the statistical data). (See 'Design versus analysis' in sect. II – 2.)

Note 1: A statistic is classified as either descriptive or inferential. A descriptive statistic summarizes/characterizes some aspect of the study experience per se, while an inferential statistic characterizes the degree to which the data are consistent with a particular model (or various particular models) for the object of study. In point of fact, however, both types of statistic are descriptive of the data, commonly representing, respectively, the study result per se and the (im)precision of this. Respective examples: an empirical rate-ratio and the width of its associated 'confidence interval.'

Note 2: Given what 'data analysis' is in epidemiological research, the term is quite a *misnomer* for the concept: at issue is *synthesis*, rather than analysis of the data. (Cf. 'Analysis and synthesis' in sect. I – 2. 2 and 'Analysis' in sect. I – 3.2.)

Decile – See 'Fractiles' (Notes 1 and 2).

Descriptive statistic – See 'Data analysis' (Note 1; and section I – 3. 2).

*Design** – Concerning the methodology of an epidemiological study, formulating the particulars of this, given the implications of the study's object design for the structure and for the empirical content in the framework of that structure. (Cf. 'Study design' in sect. II – 2.)

Note: When the object design implies that to be studied is the *etiogenesis* of an illness, to be designed is (a particular variant of) what in principle is an etiogenetic study. See 'Etiologic study.'

Design matrix – See 'Distribution matrix' (Note).

*Directionality** – "The direction of inference of a study [refs.]. It may be retrospective (backward-looking) or prospective (forward-looking)" [4].

Note 1: The 'directionality' notion in epidemiological research on etiology/etiogenesis of illness has been a *misunderstanding* – a consequence of the more proximal misunderstanding that, in this research, there are two fundamental types of study (structure/'architecture' of study) to choose between: the 'cohort study' and the 'case-control study.' Synonyms for these have been – and this is the point here – 'prospective study' and 'retrospective study,' respectively. The idea has been that in these two types of study the 'investigative movement' is, respectively, from cause to effect, prospectively, and from effect to cause, retrospectively – leaving unspecified what it is that is moving. Liberation from the cohort and trohoc fallacies would make obsolete the concept of 'directionality' associated with that malformed duality, specifically with the unworthy – and undefined – concept of 'investigative movement' these fallacies have spawned. The concept of etiology/etiogenesis of an illness is, inherently, retrospective (see sect. I – 1. 2).

Note 2: Inference based on (the evidence from) an etiologic/etiogenetic study has no 'directionality' in time; it is neither prospective nor retrospective. Instead, the 'inferential movement' is from the evidence provided by a study to the object(s) of the study, from the particularistic 'upward' to the abstract in this meaning. Inference is movement from facts (quite secure) to belief (subjective; it generally should be quite insecure).

Distribution matrix – Concerning the database of regression 'analysis,' the joint distribution of the independent variates (Xs).

Note: The particulars of the distribution matrix have great bearing on the amount of information in the database (about the parameters in the regression model, given the number of units of observation); it may have been designed to enhance the amount of information; that is, it may be a *design matrix* in this meaning.

Documentation bias – See 'Biased documentation.'

*Dummy variate** (synonym: indicator variate) – See 'Indicator variate' in section II – 2.

Note: This term is a misnomer: there is nothing dummy about an indicator variate.

Dynamic cohort – See 'Fixed and dynamic cohorts.'

*Dynamic population** (synonym: open population) – Population with turnover of membership, as it is open for exit on account of its membership being defined by a state, for the duration of that state. (Examples: residents of a given city, and policy-holders of a given system of healthcare insurance; the study population in the etiologic/etiogenetic study, involving the state of being alive, among others.)

*Efficiency** – Concerning a study, its informativeness in relation to its cost, specifically a suitable measure of the precision of the object parameter's empirical value divided by the cost of the study.

Note 1: The cost of a study is generally – and appropriately – thought of as being constituted by the 'set-up' cost followed by 'unit costs,' with the aggregate of the latter proportional to the *size* of the study; and if efficiency is defined in reference to the information-accrual following the set-up work and cost, it is independent of study size. This is a consequence of information – meaning the amount of information – being defined in the way it is defined in statistics (sect. I – 3. 2).

Note 2: For the purposes of study design it indeed is good to define efficiency in a way that makes it independent of study size; for this makes it an object of design-optimization wholly distinct from that having to do with study size. On the other hand, though, in statistical science it is more appealing to think of informativeness in terms of *standard error* (its inverse) than in those variance terms of statistics. This makes the efficiency (of a study after its set-up) a decreasing function of study size, implying *decreasing marginal efficiency with increasing size of a study*.

Note 3: The decrease in marginal informativeness with increasing size of a study (Note 2 above) is a worthy consideration in the design of the size of a study. But it is not involved in the prevailing culture of 'sample size determination.'

Note 4: In studies involving human subjects, maximization of efficiency is not only an economic desideratum but also an ethical imperative. (Cf. 'Quality of study methodology.')

*Eligibility** (synonym: admissibility) – See 'Admissibility.'

*Empirical** – Operational (as opposed to conceptual), as in 'empirical scale'; also: based directly on experience, as in 'the parameter's empirical value' (frequentist 'point estimate'); also: concerning a science or a piece of knowledge (abstract), being founded on experience (as opposed to reasoning alone, as in theoretical sciences).

Etiogenetic study (synonym: etiologic study) – See 'Etiologic study.'

*Etiologic study** (synonym: etiogenetic study) – The structure ('architecture') dictated by logic for any study of the etiology/etiogenesis of an illness (as an outgrowth of, and the necessary substitute for, its two principal precursors: the 'cohort study' and the 'case-control study'). Its elements, in reference to its *study base*, are: (1) the suitably documented case series, constituted by the entirety of the cases (as defined) occurring in the study base; (2) the similarly documented base series, derived as a fair sample of the study base; and (3) the data on these two series (of person-moments) translated into the corresponding value for the confounder-conditional rate-ratio of the occurrence of the illness in the study base, and into its associated inferential statistic(s) [9]. (Cf. 'Intervention study' in sect. III – 4 and see also 'Time'

[Notes 9 and 10] in sect. II – 3 and Note 2 under 'Analysis and synthesis' in sect. I – 2. 2.)

Note 1: In etiogenetic research, the essence of the logical structure of the study should not be viewed as a matter of study design but, instead, as an *a-priori given* (just as in the design of, say, a tennis racket the defining structure of it is a given for the design – and different from the a-priori structure of a given species of the golf-club family, say).

Note 2: The *design* of an etiogenetic study should be understood to define the particulars of the structure of the study in the framework of its a-priori, generic nature, and the way this structure with those particulars will be brought about.

Note 3: Eminent among the design challenges are these three: valid and efficient selection of the source population and the time span of its follow-up, constituting the study's source base; comprehensive identification of the cases of the illness (as defined) occurring in the source base and fair sampling of the source base; and valid documentation of both of these series in relevant regards. For, given these case and base series, suitably documented, from the source base, the rest follows without any particular challenges for design: both of these series are reduced to ones that represent (person-moments from) the actual study base (according to its operational criteria of admissibility), and the relevant statistics are derived from these. (Cf. 'Cohort fallacy' and 'Trohoc fallacy.')

Note 4: The source population may be defined indirectly, as the *catchment population* of the way case-identification is defined. See 'Source population.'

Note 5: Eminent among the design topics as for the particulars of such a study – or any study in statistical research – is commonly – but unjustifiably – taken to be its so-called sample size, meaning the *size* of the study base. (See 'Sample size determination.')

Evidence* – In epidemiological research, the product of a study; that is, the study result together with the documented genesis of this (per study design and, ultimately, the implementation of this). (Cf. sect. I – 2. 2.)

Note 1: The genesis of the study result (empirical RR, say) determines the result's validity and precision. The former is a matter of judgment (cf. 'Validity'), while the latter is subject to statistical quantification (as the result's SE or the width of its 'confidence'/imprecision interval).

Note 2: The product of an epidemiological study – even if derivative rather than original (sect. I – 2. 2) indeed is only evidence, not knowledge. It is the role of the relevant scientific community to translate the aggregate of evidence on a given object of study into knowledge about it (cf. sect. I – 2. 2). This remains ill-understood. Thus, the I.E.A. dictionary [4], under "Evidence-based public health," equates "the best available evidence" with "the most valid, precise, and relevant scientific knowledge" (as though 'evidence' and 'knowledge' were synonymous in science; cf. sect. I – 2. 2).

Expert – See 'Scientific community.'

External validity* – See 'Validity' (Notes 1 and 2).

Finding – See 'Result' (Note 2).

*Fixed cohort** – See 'Fixed and dynamic cohorts.'

Fixed and dynamic cohorts – Recent terms for muddled concepts, manifesting failure to grasp the fundamental concepts of population in epidemiological research – cohort-type (closed) population and dynamic (open) population. With understanding of these concepts, 'dynamic cohort' is seen to be a contradiction-in-terms, and also seen is that a cohort is not inherently 'fixed' in the sense of not being open to further entries (it is closed only for exits).

Fractile (synonym: quantile) – See 'Centile.'
     Note 1: As particular fractiles, the first tertile, quartile, quintile, and decile are the distribution's 33rd, 25th, 20th, and 10th centile, respectively.
     Note 2: It has become rather common to refer to an interfractile range as a fractile, as when writing about the range below the first quintile as the 'first quintile.'

*Generalizability** – See 'Validity' (Note 2).

*General population** – In epidemiological jargon, typically, the entire resident population of an administrative region (a city or a country, say), in contrast to a subpopulation of this.

Group – Concerning people, an assembly of them, rather small in number. The membership can be limited to a person-moment (as in the 'group' involved in a prevalence study). Alternatively, the membership is unlimited in prospective time (as in the intervention-specific subcohorts – 'groups' – in an RCT). A dynamic population (the study population of an etiogenetic study, say) is not a group.
     Note 1: 'Age group' is a near-routine misnomer (quite gross) for a category/range of age in reports on epidemiological studies, while, curiously, 'gender group' is not used as a term for a particular gender.
     Note 2: 'Study group' is commonly distinguished from 'control group,' including in 'case-control' studies. But insofar as distinctions are made among subgroups constituting the total group involved in a study, they all are study (sub)groups, a case-controller's 'control group' included.
     Note 3: When a group is constituted by people at particular person-moments, and especially when these person-moments are serial in time (calendar time, notably), it is natural to think, specifically, of a *series* of person-moments; and that which is common – definitional – to this series constitutes a series of that commonality. Examples: in an etiogenetic study, the case series and the base series, and the study series constituted by the two in combination. (In clinical termilogy, 'case series' is always preferred over 'case group.')

*Healthy worker effect** – "A phenomenon observed initially in studies of occupational diseases: workers often exhibit lower overall death rates than the general population, because persons who are severely ill and chronically disabled are ordinarily excluded from employment or leave employment early [ref.]" [4].

Note 1: Comparison of mortality between a cohort of workers and the local 'general population' (dynamic), though not uncommon, is a matter of strikingly primitive epidemiological research (etiogenetic). If in clinical research it would have been regarded as reasonable to study, say, the survival-enhancing efficacy of radio-therapy for a cancer by comparing mortality from the cancer between a cohort of patients and the local 'general population,' the phenomenon of 'unhealthy patient effect' would have been "observed" (in the absence of a-priori insight into the fallacy in the study design).

Note 2: Mortality in a cohort representing the index category of the causal determinant should be coupled with a *reference cohort* representing the reference category, chosen with a view to prevention of confounding. See 'Comparability' (Note 2).

*Hierarchy of evidence** – "The quality of epidemiological evidence was appraised by the Canadian Task Force on Periodic Health Examination [ref.] and the U.S. Preventive Services Task Force [ref.] as an essential prerequisite to their recommen-dations about screening and preventive interventions. The classes of evidence that these groups used are as follows:

   I: Evidence from at least one randomized controlled trial.
 II-1: Evidence from well-designed controlled trials without random allocation.
 II-2: Evidence from well-designed cohort or case-control analytic studies, prefer-ably from more than one center or research group.
 II-3: Evidence obtained from multiple time series, with or without the intervention; dramatic results in uncontrolled experiments (e.g., first use of penicillin in the 1940s) also are in this category.
  III: Opinions of respected authorities, based on clinical experience, descriptive studies, reports of expert committees, consensus conferences, etc. It is not always possible to achieve complete scientific rigor; for example, randomized controlled trials or cohort studies may be unethical or not feasible" [4].

Note 1: A study's evidentiary burden about something concerning a given generic type of object of study – some generic type of screening or intervention in the present context – is determined, jointly, by the study's characteristics in *three dimen-sions*: (1) the quality of the actual object of study (manifest in the form and domain of the study result), (2) the validity of the result of the study (per its genesis in the study's methods design and, ultimately, the execution of this), and (3) the precision of the result of the study (per the study's efficiency and size).

Note 2: A study's characteristics in the three dimensions relevant to its evi-dentiary burden cannot rationally be summarized on any *unidimensional scale* of preferability (any more than the multiple dimensions of a person's intelligence can intelligently be reduced to a unidimensional measure of intelligence).

Note 3: RCTs have no justifiable place in research on screening, nor in any other *diagnostic* research [16]. As for screening, it is knowable a priori that no early –

preclinical – diagnosis about the illness at issue can be pursued in terms other than screening. And as for research on diagnostic probability as a function of a set of diagnostic indicators, of the realizations of these, it isn't even feasible to assign particular values to these (age, e.g.).

Note 4: Evidence from a non-experimental intervention study with close adherence to the contrasted interventions (per suitable selection) and full control of confounding (given only well-documented potential confounders) is more valid than that from an RCT with poor adherence to the assigned interventions (and 'intention-to-treat' contrast). Such a non-experimental intervention study ideally has features of the etiologic/etiogenetic study [9], while the concepts of 'cohort' and 'case-control' study should be uprooted from epidemiological thought [9]. (Cf. 'Intervention study' in sect. III – 4 and 'Etiologic study,' 'Cohort fallacy,' and 'Trohoc fallacy' here).

Note 5: It presumably is inapparent to most readers what "multiple time series . . . without intervention" have to do with screening or intervention research.

Note 6: It is inapparent, too, how a study can have "dramatic results" and still be low down in the hierarchy of evidence (insofar as a hierarchy is to be conceived at all; cf. Note 2 above).

Note 7: While "opinions of respected authorities" are matters of evidence in a court of law, they do not have this status in science (cf. 'Evidence' in sect. I – 2. 2 and also here). But if they nevertheless should be viewed as the lowest level of evidence in science, and even when "based on . . . reports of expert committees, consensus conferences, etc.," then they should have this lowly status also when based on reports of such 'task forces' as are inclined to develop and/or deploy schemes for 'hierarchy of evidence' (cf. Note 2 above).

*Hill's considerations for causal inference** – See 'Causal criteria/considerations.'

*Indicator variate** – A variate indicating whether an observation falls in a particular category: 1 if yes, 0 if otherwise (cf. sect. II – 2).

Inferential statistic – See 'Data analysis' (Note 1).

Informativeness – Concerning a study, the extent to which it affords precision for the study result(s) – for the empirical value(s) of the parameter(s) at issue.

Note: A study that is highly informative in this meaning may be quite uninformative about the causality at issue. (Cf. 'Causal criteria/considerations' and 'Hypothesis testing.')

*Internal validity** – See 'Validity' (Note 1).

*Interval estimate** – Misnomer (from statistics) for a measure of the imprecision of a study result. (See 'Estimate' in sect. I – 3. 2).

*Kaplan-Meier estimate** – See 'Kaplan-Meier-Greenwood statistics' in section III – 4.

*Mantel-Haenszel estimate** – 'Estimator' of a ratio – originally odds ratio but, by extension, rate ratio also – for application with stratified data (to avoid confounding by the stratification factor[s]). The principle is this: Given that the *j*th stratum provides a numerator element n_j and a denominator element d_j, an unbiased – but inefficient – estimator of the common intra-stratum ratio is $\sum_j n_j / \sum_j d_j$. Concerning odds ratio, n_j and d_j are the two cross-products, respectively, while in the context of rate ratio they are, respectively, the numerator and denominator of the ratio of the two rates, each a product of the number of cases in one and the number of subjects (or amount of population-time) in the other. The inefficiency in this elementary formulation arises from the fact that the products, n_j and d_j, from the strata ($j = 1, 2, \ldots$) are not proportional to the respective amounts of information about the common ratio across the strata. A simple (and generally quite good) measure of information from the *j*th stratum is its size, S_j, for odds ratio the total of the cell entries in the 2×2 table, and for rate ratio the sum of the denominators. In these terms, then, the M-H estimator is $\sum_j (n_j/S_j) / \sum_j (d_j/S_j)$.

Note 1: The I.E.A. dictionary states that "The statistic may be regarded as a type of weighted average of the [stratum-specific] odds ratios," meaning the empirical values of the ORs (theoretical). This is a common misunderstanding. Only rate differences are generally amenable to (information-)weighted averaging across strata. The problem with odds ratios and rate ratios is the behavior of their (empirical) values across the strata, especially with sparse intra-stratum data: with matched pairs constituting the strata, the possible values are these four: zero, undefined (!), one, and infinity(!), as opposed to -1, 0, and 1 for the difference of proportion-type rates. Such is the genius of the M-H estimator that it functions just fine with matched pairs, even.

Note 2: The I.E.A. dictionary states that the M-H 'estimator' "can also be extended to summarization of . . . rate differences from follow-up studies." This too is untrue. Different from empirical odds ratios and rate ratios (stratum-specific), their rate-difference counterparts do not translate into that n_j/d_j form. The M-H idea is specific to stratum-specific ratios, their summarization across the strata. Rate differences are summarized by (information-)weighted averaging (cf. Note 1 above).

*Mantel-Haenszel test statistic** – Given a set of stratum-specific 2×2 tables and concern to test the null hypothesis of no association, the M-H statistic focuses, in each stratum, on a given one of the four cells – the same cell in each stratum – conditionally on the marginal totals. In the *j*th stratum this frequency has some value a_j. The marginal totals imply the null 'expected' number, E_j, in this cell and also the null variance, V_j – hypergeometric – of the number (in the sampling distribution). The statistic is, then, $\left[\sum_j (a_j - E_j) \right]^2 / \sum_j V_j$, modeled to have the chi-square distribution with one degree of freedom. (By the same token, the square root of this, with sign in accord with that of $\sum_j (a_j - E_j)$, is modeled to have the standard-Gaussian distribution.)

Note: The I.E.A. dictionary gives "Cochrane-Mantel-Haenszel" as a synonym for "Mantel-Haenszel" in the appellation of this test statistic, saying that the M-H statistic is "a slight modification of an earlier test by … Cochrane." This is not correct. The Cochrane approach addressed the 2 x 2 tables in terms of two proportions, unconditionally as for the second pairs of marginal totals. This had no role – as a starting point for "a slight modification" – in the development of the M-H statistic. The point of note is, however, that had Cochrane used unbiased, rather than ML, 'estimators' of the variances from the strata, the statistic would have been algebraically interchangeable with the M-H statistic [5, 12]. As it is, the "modification" is not always "slight": with matched pairs the Cochrane statistic is too large by a factor of two.

*Matching** – "The process of making a study group and a comparison group similar or identical with respect to their distribution of extraneous factors [refs.]. Several kinds of matching can be distinguished: *Caliper* matching … *Frequency* matching, …" [4]. (See 'Overmatching.')

Note 1: In epidemiological research on etiogenesis of illness there are, in principle, two fundamental types of matching: that of the *study base* – its reference segment to its index segment (or vice versa) – or that of the *study series* (the base series to the case series). In each, the purpose is to prevent confounding by the matching factor(s).

Note 2: In reality, though, the meaning of 'matching' in epidemiological research is, in all essence, confined to 'case-control' studies and, thus, in *the* etiologic study to selection of the base series in such a way that its distribution by the matching factors becomes identical to that of the case series (or nearly so). This matching, despite common belief to the contrary, *does not prevent confounding*. (See 'Overmatching.')

Note 3: The alternative to matched selection of the 'controls' in a 'case-control' study – to the selection of the base series in *the* etiologic study – is commonly taken to be indiscriminate selection, but this actually is but one of the alternatives; for there is a large variety of types of *discriminate* selection of the base series other than matching. The choice among them is to be made with a view to optimizing the *efficiency* of the study [5].

*Matrix** – A two-dimensional, rectangular array of quantities. (Prime example: N rows of realizations of $Y, X_1, X_2, \ldots, X_I$ in a 'data matrix' for regression 'analysis'). (See 'Design matrix' and 'Distribution matrix.')

*Meta-analysis** – Statistical synthesis of the results of original studies (distinct from 'analysis' based on the pooled data), together with production of a measure of the imprecision of the derivative result.

Note: The term is a misnomer. See 'Data analysis' (Note 2).

*Methodology** – Concerning a particular study, the aggregate of methods used. (Cf., e.g., 'Symptomatology' in sect. I – 1. 2.)

Note: Thus teaches the I.E.A. dictionary [4]: Methodology is "The scientific study of methods. The word *methodology* is all too often used when the writer means *method*."

M-H – Mantel-Haenszel.

*Multiple comparison problems** – "Problems that arise from the fact that the greater the number of conventional statistical tests of significance conducted on a data set, the greater the probability that at least one or more [*sic*] will falsely reject the null hypothesis solely because of the play of chance" [4].

Note 1: It should be understood that rejection of a null (or non-null) hypothesis is an act of a scientist's mind – a generally dubious one at that – and that it thus is not something that a statistical test of significance can do (except if, unjustifiably, taken to be a surrogate for a mind that refuses to engage in the challenging matters of scientific inference). (Cf. 'Type I and Type II errors' and 'Causal criteria/considerations' as well as 'Causal inference.')

Note 2: If multiple significance-testing on the basis of a given dataset – a single one, from a single study – indeed is a problem, then a vastly larger problem is the enormous multiplicity of such testings across separate studies – all datasets, from all epidemiological studies.

Note 3: Insofar as it indeed is taken to be a problem that the more testings get to be done, the more mistakes get to be made, the solution – the problem's obviation – on the individual level is obvious: test nothing and, perhaps better yet, be no scientist; that is, be, scientifically, an error-free nothing.

Note 4: The real problem here is not one of a dataset – that it affords and invites multiple hypothesis-testing. The real problem is the *frequentist mindset*, unequipped for scientific inference and here, exceptionally, addressing not the frequency of its errors but the cumulative number of these.

Negative confounding – Confounding that introduces a negative bias into the empirical association (RR > 1) as a measure of the effect at issue. (Cf. 'Positive confounding.')

*Negative study** – In testing a hypothesis, a study the evidence from which is generally judged as taking away from the hypothesis (i.e., from its credibility).

*Nested case-control study** – "An important type of case-control study in which cases and controls are drawn from the population in a fully enumerated cohort. . . . A set of controls is selected from subjects (i.e., noncases) at risk of developing the outcome of interest at the time of the occurrence of each case that arises in the cohort [refs.]" [4].

Note 1: Implied is a duality in types of 'case-control' study: Some 'case-control' studies are important/nested, others unimportant/unnested. But truly important to come to appreciate is that *all* proper etiogenetic studies are structured as is dictated by logic – in the form of *the* etiologic/etiogenetic study – and that this structure inherently and always is 'nested' in the *study base*. (See 'Case-control study,' Note 3, and 'Etiologic study.') Studies on etiogenesis of illness without an expressly defined study base are, well, baseless – unimportant. (Cf. 'Population-based.')

Note 2: Once it is understood that all proper etiogenetic studies are 'nested,' each within its particular study base, the challenge is to understand the general essence of these studies, as this is dictated by logic. Cases are not simply "drawn" from the study base; instead, *all* cases of the illness (as defined – typical and severe, perhaps) occurring in the study base are identified (in principle at least) for the study's case series. And given the case series, the concern in a proper etiogenetic study is not to have "controls drawn" from the study base; instead, a base series is selected so that it constitutes a fair sample of the study base. Etc. (Cf. 'Etiologic study.')

Null distribution – The distribution a particular test statistic has, according to the statistical model for this (though not necessarily in truth) in hypothetical replications of the study, conditionally on the absence of the association (descriptive) at issue. (Example: the chi-square distribution with 1 d. f. for the M-H test statistic.)

Null value – For a parameter of relation (difference or ratio, incl. regression coefficient), the value representing no relation.

*Odds ratio** – A common misnomer – along with 'relative risk' – for the result from a 'case-control' study. (At issue really is empirical incidence-density ratio, insofar as the study can be viewed as an approximation to *the* etiogenetic study [46].) (Cf. 'Etiologic study.')

Open population (synonym: dynamic population) – See 'Dynamic population.'

Operationalization – Given the occurrence relation as a result of a study's object design, translation of its elements (conceptual) into their observational counterparts in the study, and supplementation of these – in the operationalization of the study domain – by admissibility criteria of practicality and/or validity consequence. (Examples: the concept of case reduced to criteria for severe, typical case, for validity-assurance of case-identification from a directly-defined source population or of base sampling given an indirectly defined source population; histories limited to results of subject interviews without record reviews, for practicality; and domain representation limited to local residents, for practicality, and persons who are suitably compos mentis, for validity of the histories.)

OR – Odds ratio.

Outcome-probability score – See 'Propensity score.'

*Overmatching** – "An undesirable result from matching a comparison group too closely or on too many variables. Several varieties can be distinguished: 1. The matching procedure partially or completely obscures a true causal association . . . 2. The matching procedure uses . . . matching variables [that] cannot confound . . . but reduces precision. 3. The matching procedure is unduly elaborate [and] leads to difficulty in finding suitable controls" [4].

Note: The concept of overmatching actually has been that first "variety" alone, and that concept is a remarkable one in the annals of the theory of epidemiological research. In an RCT, no-one thinks of 'overblocking' – or of the typical result of randomization – with a concern about the possibility that this "partially or completely obscures the true causal association" (between outcome and the experimental intervention); and yet, if the 'controls' are closely matched to the 'cases' in a 'case-control' study (by, e.g., habit in respect to match-/light-carrying in a study of etiogenesis by smoking), the understanding has been that this "partially or completely obscures the true causal association." The remarkable thing about this has been, and even more remarkably still is, the failure to understand, or at least to suspect, the profound implication: the very concept of the 'case-control' study – the reversal in it of the natural contrast in etiogenetic research – is seriously malformed, its adoption a matter of the *trohoc fallacy*. (Cf. 'Directionality.')

*Percentile** (synonym: centile) – See 'Centile.'

Person-moment – See 'Time' (Notes 3 and 4) in section II – 3.

Point estimate – Misnomer (from statistics) for the result of a study. (See sect. I – 3. 2.)

*Population-based** – Concerning an epidemiological study (an etiologic one, typically), the quality of having an expressly defined population as the referent of its result. (Most commonly meant is a particular 'general population.')
    Note: Implied by the use (proud) of this term is that not all epidemiological studies are based on the experience of a defined population. This indeed is commonly true about 'case-control' studies on etiogenesis, but most unfortunate. All epidemiological studies should be based on defined study populations – without regarding these as 'target' populations of the studies (scientific). In the framework of *the* etiogenetic study, at issue operationally is the definition of the *source population* – indirectly, as the catchment population for the cases, if not directly.

Population-time – See 'Time' in section II – 3.
    Note: A series of person-moments (as the referent of a rate of prevalence, say) is a degenerate case of population-time.

Positive confounding – Confounding that introduces a positive bias into the empirical association ($RR > 1$) as a measure of the effect at issue. (Cf. 'Negative confounding.')

Positive study – In testing a hypothesis, a study the evidence from which is generally judged to support the hypothesis (i.e., to enhance its credibility).

*Power** – See section I – 3. 2 and 'Sample size determination' below.
    Note: The concept of a study's 'power' should be replaced by that of the *precision* of its result.

*Precision** (synonym: reproducibility) – See 'Accuracy and precision.'

Prevention of confounding – Seeing to it that the study base will be unconfounded by a particular potential confounder (or a set of these). (Cf. Note 5 under 'Confounding,' and 'Control of confounding.')

Note: In etiologic/etiogenetic research, the principal means to prevent confounding is formation of the *causal contrast* in the object of study in such a way that the potential confounder's distributions in the index and reference segments of the study base are essentially similar. See 'Healthy worker effect' (Note 2) here, and 'Quality of study object(s)' (#4 under it) in section III – 3.

Primary base – A study base resulting from defining the source population directly (as distinct from indirectly, secondary to direct definition of how cases of the illness are identified). (Cf. 'Secondary base' and see 'Source population.')

Propensity score* – Confounder score addressing the probability of the cause – rather than the outcome.
Note: Subsequent to the introduction of that pair of confounder scores [45], both of them addressing probabilities – propensities, that is – the term 'propensity score' has been introduced with reference only to the cause. 'Cause-probability score' would be a more apposite term – distinct from 'outcome-probability score.'

Prospective* – See 'Time' (Notes 8, 10, and 12) in section II – 3 and 'Cohort study.'

Protocol* – For an epidemiological (or a meta-epidemiological clinical) study, the document that specifies the component actions and sequences of these in the execution of the study design.

Publication bias* – See 'Bias' (Note 6).

Quality of study methodology – That which is the concern to 'optimize' – maximize – in the design of the methods of a study (epidemiological), given the design of the object of the study. (Cf. 'Quality of study object[s]' in sect. II – 3.)
Note 1: In studying the etiology/*etiogenesis* of an illness – which is what epidemiological research mostly is about – the quality of the design of the methods of study – of the study proper – is first a matter of certain requirements of *validity* – of validity assurance.
Note 2: Even though the investigators presume the study base to be free of *selection bias*, for the purpose of validity assurance in the relevant scientific community they are supposed to report the spatio-temporal particulars of the study base. (Those experts may not agree about the freedom from selection bias.)
Note 3: Another one of the component requirements is freedom from *documentation bias* resulting from (1) valid operationalization of the elements (theoretical) in the designed occurrence relation (incl. its domain criteria), defining the RR parameter(s) being studied; (2) a valid pair of study series resulting from valid identification of the case series together with valid sampling for the base series; and (3) valid conditioning of the empirical RR, in reference to what was intended by the study's object design.
Note 4: *Residual confounding* affecting the study result is a consequence of deficient methods design only insofar as the conditionality (of the empirical RR)

designed into the object of study was not assured by the study's methods design. Otherwise an incomplete conditioning (of the empirical RR) is a defect in the study's object design.

Note 5: That a study be designed to make its *efficiency* as high as possible is an economic desideratum; and more importantly, in experimental studies it also is an ethical imperative. (Cf. 'Institutional Review Board' in sect. III – 4.)

Note 6: One of the determinants of the efficiency of an etiogenetic study has to do with the choice of the *study base*. Most efficient is, of course, the use of a pre-existing database. Otherwise, a local study-base is generally more efficient than a distant one, and so also is one with relatively great variability of the etiogenetic histories, notably in the sense of relative commonality of both the index history and the reference history.

Note 7: Another one of the determinants of the efficiency of such a study is the *mode of sampling* of the study base. The broadest choice is between indiscriminate and discriminate – stratified – sampling. A special case of the latter is sampling so as to make the base series matched to the case series. (Such matching, by confounders, does not, generally, optimize the efficiency of the mode of sampling; and such matching is altogether irrelevant for the attainment of control of confounding. Cf. 'Matching.')

Note 8: Yet another determinant of note regarding the efficiency of an etiogenetic study is the *size ratio* between the case and base series. (Optimal is the inverse of the square root of the corresponding unit-cost ratio.)

Note 9: A study's *size* is a matter of quantity rather than quality, and so, as a consequence, also is a study's (degree of) *precision*/informativeness.

Quartile – See 'Fractile' (Notes 1 and 2).

Quasi-rate – A quantity of the form of a rate (empirical) but involving, in lieu of the size of the rate's referent, only a sample frequency as a (stochastically) proportional representation of the size of this referent.

Note: Quasi-rates are a central feature of the etiologic/etiogenetic/etiognostic study – and also of the deployment of this as a paradigm for the prognostic study (cf. Note 3 under 'Prognostic study' in sect. III – 4 .)

Quintile – See 'Fractile' (Notes 1 and 2).

Randomization – See 'Randomized controlled trial' in section III – 4.

*Randomized controlled trial** – See section III – 4.

*Rare-disease assumption** – In 'case-control' studies, the notion that the obtained result – thought to be odds ratio – coincides with 'relative risk' if, and only if, the illness is rare.

Note: This 'assumption' has been a misunderstanding [46], as has by now become quite commonly understood.

RCT – Randomized controlled trial.

Regression analysis* – See 'General linear model' (Notes 3 and 4) in section I – 3. 2.

Note 1: The *process* meaning of the term is: Fitting a regression model – commonly a general or generalized linear model – to a set of statistical/numerical data – to obtain fitted/empirical values of the parameters – and deriving measures of the precisions of these, commonly their standard errors. The 'analysis' may be extended to, for example, assessment of goodness of fit or adjustment for overparametrization/overfitting; see 'Shrinkage' in section III – 4.

Note 2: 'Analysis' is a misnomer in this context. (See 'Analysis' in sect. I – 2. 2.)

Relative risk* – See 'Attributable and relative risk' (Note in particular).

Replication distribution – The distribution a parameter's empirical value has – according to the statistical model for this (though not necessarily in truth) – in hypothetical replications of the study, infinite in number, with the same design in all relevant regards, including in respect to efficiency and size.

Representative sample* – A sample typical of the sampled set of objects (e.g., person-moments in study base).

Note: 'Simple' – distinct from 'stratified' – random sampling produces a stochastically representative sample. A stratified random sample is stochastically representative within the strata of sampling.

Reproducibility* (synonym: precision) – See 'Accuracy and precision.'

Residual confounding* – The confounding in the result of a study on causality (etiogenetic, most notably), reflecting incomplete prevention and/or control of confounding.

Result – In an epidemiological study, the empirical counterpart of the object (theoretical) of a study. (Cf. 'Evidence.')

Note 1: Specifically, in an epidemiological study (original or derivative), the result is constituted by the empirical value(s) of the parameter(s) constituting the object(s) of study. Example: From a study to test an etiogenetic hypothesis, the result generally is an empirical rate-ratio conditional on some confounders.

Note 2: Seriously *misleading terminology* permeates epidemiologists' writing – and public speaking – about the results of epidemiological studies to test etiogenetic hypotheses. The result is commonly said to be the 'relative risk' that the study 'found' or 'showed,' the RR value said to mean RR-fold 'increased risk' – characterized as 'significant' to boot. But: if a person tosses 10 coins by left hand and another 10 by right hand, and if the respective rates of heads turn out to be 8/10 and 2/10 ($P < 0.01$), it is not true that the relative risk of heads with a left-hand toss was four-fold relative to that with a right-hand toss in this experience (only the empirical RR was); left-hand toss did not mean increased risk of heads, much less a significant one; and overall, nothing was shown or found – even when having no bias or confounding to consider. (Cf. 'Hypothesis testing.')

Retrospective* – See 'Time' (Notes 8, 9, and 12) in section II – 3 and 'Case-control study.'

RR – Rate ratio (empirical).

Sample size – See 'Size of study.'

Sample size determination* – "The mathematical process [sect. 1 – 3. 2] of deciding, before a study begins, how many subjects should be studied. The factors to be taken into account include the incidence or prevalence of the condition being studied, the estimated or putative relationship among the variables in the study, the power that is desired, and the maximum allowable magnitude of Type I error" [4].

   Note 1: Otherwise phrased, study-size determination is the *translation* into the corresponding study size the *givens* in terms of (the determinants of) the study's efficiency and the intended degree of the study's informativeness; determined is the size that should be adopted for the study if the premises pertaining to efficiency are correct and correctly translated into the study's efficiency, and the particular degree of informativeness actually is optimal to produce – not too low, nor too high.

   Note 2: Of particular note is that a-priori commitment to a particular degree of informativeness, and this, notably, with no "mathematical process of deciding" what this degree of informativeness ought to be, so as not to be too low or too high.

   Note 3: Actually, that "mathematical process" is but the first phase in the design of the size of an epidemiological study. A second phase generally is carried out by peer reviewers of the grant application for the study. In this phase the process is not a matter of judging the correctness of the premises of the first-phase determination of the study's size and possible recalculation based on changed premises of that kind. Altogether *non-mathematical*, this second-stage determination of a study's size commonly amounts to setting it to zero (and corresponding adjustment of the budget for the study [12]).

   Note 4: The indisputable fact that this second phase thoroughly trumps the first phase should have been seen, long ago already, to be a very persuasive indication of the speciousness of that "mathematical process of deciding ... how many subjects should be studied." But, as R. H. Brown notes in his *Man and the Stars* (1978), "Anyone who has read the trial of Galileo knows that human institutions tend to preserve ideas as rock preserves fossils." One of those institutions, by this example among others – such as the ideas of 'cohort study' and 'case-control study' – evidently is the I.E.A.

Scientific community – Given evidence – notably derivative evidence (sect. I – 2. 2) – on an object of epidemiological research, the aggregate of experts on its translation into knowledge (updated) on the object of study.

Note 1: An expert as a member of the topic-relevant scientific community of epidemiologists is characterized by unsurpassed extra-epidemiological knowledge about, and related to, the topic at issue, and also full familiarity with all of the published epidemiological research on it; and besides, (s)he masters the principles of the relevant genre of epidemiological research, including those of inference from it. Beyond these 'technical' qualifications, (s)he has an unbiased, impartial attitude about the topic.

Note 2: Two aggregates of persons generally unqualified to engage in the inference involved in the translation of evidence into justifiable subjective belief, even, are these: the investigators involved in the study (derivative, perhaps) and the practitioners of 'evidence-based medicine' (whether clinical or community medicine). The investigators generally lack the requisite impartial attitude, and those practitioners generally lack the requisite expertise.

SE – See section I – 3. 2.

Secondary base – A study base resulting from defining the source population indirectly (as the catchment population of the way cases of the illness are identified). (Cf. 'Primary base' and see 'Source population.')

Selection bias* – See 'Biased base' (Note 2).

Simple random sampling – Probability sampling with the same probability for each member of the sampled set of units. (Cf. 'Stratified random sampling.')

Size of study – The amount of population-time or the number (finite) of person-moments constituting the study base; also: the number of cases of the illness occurring in the study base (given a substantially larger base series).

Note: A study's size and its efficiency jointly determine the precision of its result.

Source population – The population (open or closed) in the time-course of which the study population is defined or formed.

Note 1: For an etiogenetic study the *study* population – being open/dynamic – can generally be only defined (within the source population), without it being subject to being (operationally) formed. (Cf. Note 3 under 'Etiologic study.') For an intervention study, by contrast, the study population can be, and is, formed within the time-course of the source population (ultimately by the act of enrolment into the study cohort).

Note 2: The source population's *definition is either direct or indirect.* In the context of an etiogenetic study, direct definition may be given to the way in which the cases (for the first-stage case series, before the reduction of this to the ultimate case series) are identified. This is tantamount to defining the source population as the *catchment population* of this manner of case-identification. This population is dynamic, one whose members, at any given moment, are in the 'were-would' state of: were the outcome event to occur at this moment, it would be identified for the study's first-stage series of cases.

*Standard population** – In standardization of rates, the population (possibly only hypothetical) whose structure – distribution – according to the person-characterizers at issue (commonly age and gender) provides the 'standard' – meaning shared – weights for the strata. (See 'Rate' in sect. I – 1. 2, Notes 6 and 7.)

*Standardized rate** – See 'Rate' (Notes 6 and 7) in section 1. 2.

*Statistical significance** – "The probability of the observed or a larger value of a test statistic under the null hypothesis. Often equivalent to the probability of the observed or larger degree of association under the null hypothesis. This usage is synonymous with P-value" [4]. (Cf. 'P-value.')

Note 1: Recently, Stang et alii [47] wrote this: "the tyranny of [statistical] significance testing is still highly prevalent in biomedical literature, even after decades of warnings against [it; ref.]. ... An important way out of the significance fallacies ... is to interpret statistical findings based on confidence intervals that convey both the size and precision of estimated effect measures." This was seconded in an adjoining, invited Commentary by Rothman [48], who wrote that statistical significance-testing is "a flawed approach" that "should have been discarded long ago [in favor of reliance] on estimation using confidence intervals."

Note 2: Those authors echo, for example, Ziliak and McCloskey, who wrote that "statistical significance should be a tiny part of an inquiry concerned with the size and importance of relationships. Unhappily it has become the central and standard error of many sciences. ... Real science depends on size, on magnitude" [49].

Note 3: Statistical significance-testing – in the meaning of producing the null P-value – is the usual final element of *hypothesis-testing in statistical science*, specifically in the usual frequentist framework of statistical thought in this. Rather than objecting to frequentism in this, these abolitionists are saying that hypothesis-testing – which they equate with statistical significance-testing – has no justifiable place in statistical science, that it should be replaced by focus on quantification of parameters of Nature.

Note 4: Those abolitionists are failing to appreciate, for one, that in science one is supposed to take all parameters of relation/difference (incl. association measures of effect) to have the value that corresponds to absence of the relation/difference till there is good reason to think otherwise – on the basis of the evidence from hypothesis-testing, if not a priori. (Cf. Note 2 under 'Hypothesis' in sect. I – 2. 2).

Note 5: A more subtle but equally important point, also missed by those abolitionists, has to do with the very magnitudes they are concerned to focus on, in lieu of hypothesis-testing. While in the null situation the parameter at issue has a single (the null) value in all subdomains of the domain of study, the hypothesized non-null situation does not share this simplicity. The parameter at issue – etiogenetic rate-ratio, most notably – cannot be presumed to have a single non-null value, and therefore the advocated type of quantification – addressing a single value for the parameter (usually rate ratio) – is targeted at something that actually is a mere phantasm. (Cf. Note 5 under 'Causal rate-ratio' in sect. II – 3.)

Note 6: Criticism of testing statistical significance (in statistical science) – once this is the topic – should begin with the way the null P-value is conceptualized by the abolitionists, like others (i.e., as a probability rather than as a statistic with particular distributional properties; cf. 'P-value'). An appropriate broader criticism would be that the null P-value should be viewed jointly with the result on the parameter at issue (RR, notably), the credibility of this as representation of the parameter's theoretical value conditionally on the hypothesis being true [12].

Note 7: All in all, thus, hypothesis-testing must be understood to deserve an eminent role in epidemiological research (on etiogenesis of illness, notably), and the precision of the result of a hypothesis-testing study can very well be expressed by the null P-value as a supplement to the empirical value of the parameter at issue. The result together with the null P-value imply the entire P-value function and, thus, whichever measure of the result's precision (width of the 95% 'confidence'/imprecision interval, notably). (Entertained in this is single-valued non-null situation across the subdomains represented in the study base, without the specificity that is necessary in scientific quantification.)

*Stochastic** – Involving the vagaries of chance. (Example: 'stochastic' representativeness of a simple random sample.)

*Stratified random sampling** – Probability sampling separately for a set of strata of the sampled set of units, with a view to efficiency in gaining information about some overall unstratified parameter descriptive of the overall set of sampled units. (Cf. 'Simple random sampling.')

*Study base** – In an epidemiological study (scientific), the aggregate of population-time or the series of person-moments for which the outcome's rate of occurrence is documented.

Note 1: The study base is the *referent* of the result of a study.

Note 2: When the study base is an aggregate of population-time, the first-order result is about incidence density (as a function of its determinants); for prognostic purposes it is to be translated into the cumulative incidence it implies [16].

Note 3: When the study base is a series of person-moments, the result can be one of prevalence (its rate as a function of determinants of this); but, alternatively, it can be one of incidence (concerning a very short-term outcome, so that the details of its timing don't matter, nor are there opportunities for the follow-up's termination before the outcome's realization).

Note 4: Whereas the documented occurrence of the outcome takes place in the study base, the determinants may well (and commonly do) have their referents in times when the persons were not yet contributing to the study base.

Study group – The 'group' of 'cases' in a 'case-control' study of etiology/etiogenesis; also: the group of focal interest. (Example: in an intervention trial, the intervention/index group, rather than the control/reference group.)

Note: Actually, all subgroups in a study constitute, jointly, the overall study group. (Cf. 'Study population.')

Study population – The population (open or closed) the time-course of which constitutes the population-time of the study base; also: the population in the time-course of which the series (finite) of person-moments are arrested for constituting the study base.

Note: For an etiologic/etiogenetic study, the study population generally is open, *dynamic*. This is the case even when the source population is closed, a cohort. For, membership is based on the *state* – transient state – represented by the study domain (being alive, etc.).

Study time – See 'Time' (Notes 7 and 8) in section II – 3.

*Systematic error** – Bias in the result of a study consequent to bias in the methodology of the study.

T_0 – The zero point of a scale of time. (See 'Time' in sect. II – 3.)

*Target population** – In epidemiological research, a concept associated with a funda-mental misunderstanding, confusing scientific research with sample surveys: "The ideal epidemiological study would be based on probability samples from a very large population in order to permit generalization from the study group to the larger population with specifiable limits of precision" [2].

Note: No-one in a toxicological or pharmacological laboratory dreams of a prob-ability sample of a very large population of newborn albino mice or whatever other type of animal for a causality-oriented experiment. Nor do clinical researchers designing an RCT dream of a probability sample of a very large population of persons eligible for participation in the trial.

Tertile – See 'Fractile' (Notes 1 and 2).

Test-based confidence interval – 'Confidence interval' deduced from two other points of the P-value function: the null point (to which corresponds the null P-value) and the 'point estimate' (to which corresponds P = 0.50). With RR the empirical value ('point estimate') of rate ratio, and g the realization of a standard-Gaussian test statistic corresponding to the null P-value, the test-based 95% limits for the theoretical RR are [12, 46], on the log scale,

$$\log(RR) [1 \mp 1.96/g];$$

and if RD is the empirical rate difference, then, correspondingly, the 95% limits are [12, 46]

$$(RD) [1 \mp 1.96/g].$$

Note 1: When the null P-value (one-sided) is 0.025, one of the limits is to be the parameter's null value (RR = 1, RD = 0). These test-based limits satisfy this requirement.

Note 2: These limits for RR have the 'point estimate' as their geometric mean, while the limits for RD have the 'point estimate' as their arithmetic mean. These properties are near-ubiquitous for 'interval estimates' used in epidemiological research at present. Implied is a model according to which the variance of the empirical value of log(RR), and of RD, is constant over the range of the interval (i.e., independent of the parameter's value in this range).

Note 3: To the extent that this constant-variance modeling is not realistic, used should be limit-specific variances; and this need is, generally, much more compelling for the proximal one of the limits, the one closer to the parameter's null value. It deserves note that if the null P-value is correct, so also is the test-based limit coinciding with the null P-value (cf. Note 1 above); and it also deserves note that null variance is involved in all first-principles test statistics, such as the M-H chi-square statistic (different from the involvement of SE in Wald-type test statistics).

Note 4: For the epidemiologically so important etiologic/etiogenetic proportion/fraction – empirically (RR – 1) / RR for those with a positive history for the cause at issue; and for a population, this proportion multiplied by the prevalence of the positive history [24] – the test-based limits correspond to those of the RR.

Trohoc fallacy – See 'Case-control study' (Note 3).

*Type I and Type II errors** – In frequenstist-type testing of an epidemiological hypothesis (conjecturing that a specified relation obtains), Type I error is rejection of the corresponding 'null hypothesis' if it is (substantively) correct, while Type II error is acceptance of the 'null hypothesis' when it is (substantively) incorrect.

Note: These errors should be non-existent in epidemiological research, consequent to proper conception of an epidemiological study per se and of inference on the basis of it. (See 'Study' in sect. I – 2. 2, 'Estimate' and 'Inference' in sect. I – 3. 2, and 'Etiologic study' here as well as – and especially – 'Hypothesis testing' in sect. II – 2.)

*Validation** – Demonstration of validity (unbiasedness) or making valid (by removing bias).

Note: An important example of validation is what statisticians term *cross-validation* in the context of regression analysis with overparametrization/overfitting; and an important example of this is 'shrinkage' by means of the 'leave-out-one' method. (See 'Shrinkage in sect. III – 4.)

*Validity** – Unbiasedness; that is, freedom from bias.

Note 1: Insofar as a distinction is to be made between 'internal' and 'external' validity (à la I.E.A. dictionary), *internal validity* must be taken to be freedom from documentation bias in respect to a descriptive result, and from confounding bias besides in respect to (what is presented as) a causal result; and *external validity* must be taken to be internal validity together with freedom from selection bias, that is, overall validity.

Note 2: External validity is generally conceptualized as *generalizability* (incl. in the I.E.A. dictionary). Different concepts of generalization and generalizability are presented in section I – 2. 2.

PART III
META-EPIDEMIOLOGICAL CLINICAL RESEARCH

III – 1. INTRODUCTION

There is no generally agreeable – objective – way to define the scope of *clinical research* in the general framework of medical research, commonly taken to encompass 'basic' and 'applied' medical research. The prevailing textbook-definitions of clinical research are, accordingly, highly variable; and they are in various other ways untenable besides [16].

But just as in the framework of epidemiological research, it is possible to identify the most important, quintessentially 'applied' genre of clinical research. This is research to advance the *knowledge-base* of clinical medicine, of scientific clinical medicine. It thus is research to develop the general (abstract-general) knowledge-base for setting gnostic – dia-, etio-, and prognostic – probabilities. Needed to this end is research on *gnostic probability functions* [16].

Preeminent in the needed research is study of diagnostic probabilities as functions (descriptive) of diagnostic indicators, and of prognostic probabilities as functions of prognostic indicators (descriptively) jointly with choice of intervention (causally) and prognostic time. Etiognostic clinical research is less eminent a topic, with probability functions for iatrogenesis of illness (or mere sickness) deserving the highest priority in this. Remarkably, advancement of the knowledge-base of clinical etiognosis (about iatrogenesis) has not yet emerged as the principal mission in epidemiologists' 'pharmaco-epidemiology.'

The needed diagnostic research is challenging because of the need to ascertain, in each of the person-moments in the study series/base, the truth about the presence/absence of the illness at issue. The prognostic research, by contrast, can be based on data now routinely collected in randomized trials on interventions [9, 16].

III – 2. INTRODUCTORY TERMS AND CONCEPTS

See note opening section II – 2.

CEA – Cost-effectiveness analysis.

Clinical research/study – The I.E.A. dictionary [4] defines *clinical study* as, "An investigation involving persons and aiming to understand or control disease and other health states in persons. Often – but not exclusively – carried out on patients, by physicians, and in a health care setting. Problems found worthy of investigation in caring for patients are frequently taken to the laboratories; yet the nature and purpose of the investigation often remains clinical, and the laboratory results must be tested again on actual persons – eventually by integrating epidemiological and statistical reasoning with clinical, pathophysical, and microbiological (e.g., genetic) reasoning [ref.]."

Note 1: Other examples of recent definitions, specifically of *clinical research*, include these [16]:

1. "Foremost among [the clinical sciences] is clinical epidemiology … the science of making predictions about individual patients by counting clinical events in groups of similar patients and using strong scientific methods to ensure that the predictions are accurate" [50].
2. "This book is about the science of doing clinical research in all of its forms: translational research, clinical trials, patient-oriented research, epidemiologic research, behavioral science and health services research" [51].
3. "[S]ome researchers have narrowly defined clinical research to refer to clinical trials … , while others have … even include[d] animal studies, the results of which more or less directly apply to humans. … I have chosen to adopt a 'middle-of-the-road' definition … research conducted with human subjects (or material of human origin) for which the investigator directly interacts with the human subjects at some point during the study" [52].
4. "The purpose of this book is to teach both the 'users' and 'doers' of quantitative clinical research. Principles and methods of clinical epidemiology are used to obtain quantitative evidence on diagnosis, etiology, and prognosis of disease and on effects of interventions" [53].

O. S. Miettinen, *Epidemiological Research: Terms and Concepts*, 139
DOI 10.1007/978-94-007-1171-6_9, © Springer Science+Business Media B.V. 2011

Note 2: Evidently, just as with epidemiological research, there is no objective – generally agreed-upon – definition of clinical research; very far from it. But just as it is feasible to define *quintessentially applied* epidemiological research (cf. sect. II – 2), it is feasible to define – quite objectively – its counterpart in clinical research: research intended to serve advancement of the (scientific) *knowledge-base* of clinical medicine – of the knowledge base of gnosis in clinical medicine [16]. (Cf. sect. III – 1.) This research is *meta-epidemiological*, as it addresses rates of occurrence of phenomena of health but not for the advancement of epidemiology (its practice). Its aim is advancement of the knowledge-base of clinical medicine (its practice) – by the development of rates-based gnostic probability functions (16).

Note 3: A reasonable definition of clinical research at large might be: Research intended to advance, potentially at least, clinical medicine (its practice, incl. in terms other than its knowledge-base; [16]). (Cf. 'Epidemiological research' in sect. II – 2.)

*Clinical study** – See 'Clinical research/study.'

*Cost-effectiveness analysis** – See 'Outcomes research' (Notes 5 and 6).

*Cox regression** – Regression 'analysis' of RCT data under the proportional hazards model, to address hazard ratio. (See 'Proportional hazards model.')

Note: There now is an epidemiology-inspired alternative to Cox regression for use with RCT data [9]. See 'Prognostic study' in section III – 4.

*Effectiveness** (synonym: efficacy) – See 'Efficacy.'

Effectiveness research (synonym: outcomes research) – See 'Outcomes research' (Note 2).

*Efficacy** (synonym: effectiveness) – See section I – 1. 2. (Cf. 'Safety.')

Note 1: According to the I.E.A. dictionary, *efficacy* is: "The extent to which a specific intervention, procedure, regimen, or service produces a beneficial result under ideal conditions; the benefit or utility to the individual or the population of the service, treatment regimen, or intervention. Ideally, the determination of efficacy is based on the results of a randomized controlled trial."

Note 2: According to the I.E.A. dictionary, "In the usage made common among epidemiologists by Archibald L. Cochrane (1909-1988) and others, [*effectiveness*] is a measure of the extent to which a specific intervention, procedure, regimen, or service, when deployed in the field in the usual circumstances, does what it is intended to do, for a specified population [ref.]. A measure of the extent to which a health care intervention fulfills its objectives in practice."

Note 3: What Cochrane actually said (on p. 2 of the booklet [54] referenced in the quote above), when contemplating the efficiency – cost-effectiveness – of the U.K. National Health Service, is this:

It is in this sense [of using an RCT "to measure the effect of a particular medical action in altering the natural history of a particular disease for the better"] that I use the word 'effective,' ... and I use it in relation to research results, as opposed to the results obtained when therapy is applied in routine clinical practice in a defined community. Some people would like to use the word 'efficacious' [i.e., having efficacy] for this ... but as I dislike the word I have not used it here. ... Different strategies of management may be needed ["in the community"] to achieve levels of effectiveness comparable to those reached in the RCTs. ... To cover all these varied activities I have used the word 'efficacy.' I would agree that it is not a very satisfactory index. It might, for instance, benefit from being further subdivided into its component parts. ... I hope that others will deal with this neglected subject in the future ...

Clearly, Cochrane was not responsible for the distinction epidemiologists now commonly make between efficacy and effectiveness (cf. Note 2 above), while medicine generally does not (sect. I – 2. 2).

Note 4: Given that Cochrane is being held in very high regard, by 'clinical epidemiologists' in particular, note is to be taken of what he actually said. For one, *effectiveness* he evidently took to be synonymous with 'efficaciousness,' a cognate of 'efficacy,' and he had a linguistic preference for the 'effectiveness.' And by 'effectiveness' he meant that which is addressed in *RCTs*! (Cf. Note 2 above.)

Note 5: Cochrane did not say, nor even insinuate, that RCTs represent "ideal conditions" (Note 1 above) and are, thereby, of limited relevance in regard to "the field," to the "usual circumstances" there (Note 2 above). What he said, instead, is that the degree of efficacy/effectiveness manifest in RCTs is to be the goal "in the community" as well, and that "strategies of management" different from those in RCTs "may be needed to achieve this goal." He naturally was interested, in principle, in the efficacy – efficaciousness, effectiveness – of "these varied activities" in providing for the interventions addressed in RCTs, for reaping the RCT-measured benefits of the interventions. He did not think it would be "satisfactory" to address "these varied activities" as non-specific aggregates jointly with the actual interventions as to efficacy. He saw the need to address separately the "component parts" involved in these aggregates – the RCT-measured benefits a central one among the components.

Note 6: The American Heritage dictionary presents as synonyms the words 'effective,' 'efficacious,' and 'effectual.' The notion that these words denote different concepts actually emerged from the Office of Technology Assessment of the U. S. Congress (see 'Outcomes research').

Expert system – See section I – 1. 2.

*False negative/positive** – See section I – 1. 2.

*Hazard** – Concerning risk as a function of the time that is involved in its definitions (as cumulative probability over time) for various spans of time, the probability density of this (as a function of that time).

Note 1: Like risk, hazard (time-specific) is a parameter (of Nature), not a statistic.

Note 2: 'Hazard' in this meaning is terminology of statisticians. The epidemiological term is *incidence density*.

Hazard ratio – In Cox regression, the ratio of two hazards, each of these corresponding to a possible realization of one of the independent variates. (See 'Proportional hazards model.')

Health-related quality of life – See 'Outcomes research' (Notes 4-6).

HR – Hazard ratio (this parameter, distinct from an 'estimate' of it).

HRQL – Health-related quality of life.

Indication – Realization of an indicator.

Indicator – A person-characterizer that gives, by its realization, an indication of a person's health – a diagnostic, etiognostic, or prognostic indication (the indication constituting an element in the gnostic profile of the case).
    Note 1: *Diagnostic* indicators fall in two principal categories: risk indicators and manifestational indicators (both discriminating between/among the differential-diagnostic possibilities).
    Note 2: *Etiognostic* indicators are modifiers of the causal/etiogenetic rate-ratio.
    Note 3: *Prognostic* indicators are risk indicators for the adverse event/state at issue in the prognosis. Intervention is a prognostic factor (causal), prognosis being conditional on the choice of intervention.

Meta-epidemiological clinical research – Research that is epidemiological in form but clinical in substance, aimed at advancement of the knowledge-base of (the practice of) clinical medicine. (Cf. 'Epidemiological research' in sect. II – 2 and 'Clinical research/study,' Note 2.)

*Outcome** – See section II – 2.

*Outcomes research** – "Research on outcomes of interventions. This is a large part of the work of clinical epidemiologists and epidemiologists involved in health services research" [4].
    Note 1: Given that outcomes research is "research on outcomes of interventions," the term is synonymous with 'intervention research' and 'intervention-prognostic research.' It needs to be Ockham's-razored out of the lexicons of epidemiology.
    Note 2: The term 'outcomes research' was adduced by the Office of Technology Assessment of the U. S. Congress [55], now closed. Technologies to the OTA encompassed entities such as "drugs" (instead of pharmaco-interventions) and diagnostics; and the OTA quite cavalierly adopted the notion that *diagnostics*, too, are invoked to change the course of health for the better – that their use, too, is intervention. Medical outcomes research thus was, to the OTA, research to study

the effectiveness of both diagnostics and treatments. In its final report [56], as it was being closed by the Congress, the OTA recast outcomes research as *effectiveness research*. The OTA notion that use of diagnostics is intervention, supposed to have health-enhancing effectiveness, was embraced by the leadership of American radiology [57, 58] and even by the U. S. National Cancer Institute [59].

Note 3: It was the OTA that adduced the notion that a distinction is to be made between 'efficacy' and 'effectiveness' [55], and this has been embraced by epidemiologists – with false attribution to A. L. Cochrane (cf. 'Efficacy.')

Note 4: Integral to the concept of a medical intervention's effectiveness naturally is the course of health that the intervention is intended to change; and to this the OTA's 'outcomes research' ideology brought the innovative notion that measures of *health-related quality of life* are to be included among the outcomes. This, too, has been embraced by epidemiologists – even though the clinical idea has been that the patient-relevant effects of interventions have to do with sickness (discomfort, dysfunctionality, deformity) along with survival, and that the disutility of sickness isn't really a matter of medicine but, instead, one of *subjective valuation not subject to general medical knowledge* (from intervention research). But the idea was, specifically, that HRQL should be assessed in each piece of 'outcomes research.' A more rational idea is that were HRQL to be subject to research – psychological [60] – the research should address various types of sickness and independently of the effects (medical) on sickness.

Note 5: Central in the OTA's concerns about medical interventions was 'cost-effectiveness analysis,' CEA, of these; and central to this, in turn was taken to be an intervention's effectiveness in terms of its resultant gain in *'quality-adjusted life years,'* QALYs. For this measure, HRQL is defined on a (quantitative) scale in which "1 corresponds to perfect health and ... 0 corresponds to a health state judged equivalent to death" [61]. The scientific physician's intellect faces a serious challenge attempting to apprehend the concept of HRQL that is "equivalent to death," and equally if actually meant is that HRQL = 0 characterizes a person's life post mortem!

Note 6: Puzzling also is the CEA idea that appropriate to consider is an intervention's effect of QALYs in terms of the *average* – statisticians' 'expected value' – of this across the persons that might be treated. For, with or without the intervention, a particular patient faces a probability distribution for the remaining amount of QALYs; and while only one of these potential amounts of QALYs will materialize, this amount will not be the 'expected' one, the probability-weighted average of the possible ones. Rational people – 'decision analysts' included – could well opt for an intervention that reduces the 'expected' amount of remaining QALYs – just as they buy insurance well aware that at issue is a monetary transaction with negative 'expected' result (monetary) for them (different from the insurance company).

Note 7: As perhaps is evident from the ideas underpinning and surrounding 'outcomes research,' epidemiological and clinical researchers should not uncritically adopt concepts – nor terms such as 'outcomes research' – originating outside their own circles. And even more important is critical reflection on the *principles* of intervention research that are introduced from the outside: The OTA in its last report on 'outcomes research' – which it in that context renamed 'effectiveness research' (cf. above) – remarked on the congressional stipulation that effectiveness is to be studied "in ordinary circumstances, in ordinary settings" as distinct from RCTs; it said that heeding this stipulation has been the "signal failure" of the implementation of the OTA's ideas by the U. S. Government's Agency for Health Care Policy and Research (now Agency for Health Care Research and Quality).

*Proportional hazards model** – The model for Cox regression:

$$H = \left[\exp \left(\sum_i B_i X_i \right) \right] H_0,$$

where H is hazard and H_0 is H conditional on $X_i = 0$ for all i.

Note: Based on two possible realizations of X_i, the corresponding *hazard ratio* is the ratio of the respective values of H conditional on the same set of values for the other Xs. It thus is the exponential of the $B_i X_i$ difference between those two values of X_i. (If the model involves no product terms with X_i, HR = exp$[B_i]$.)

*Quality-adjusted life year** – See 'Outcomes research' (Note 5).

QALY – Quality-adjusted life year.

Technology assessment – See 'Outcomes research' (Notes 2-7).

Theory of clinical medicine – Concepts, principles, and terminology of clinical medicine (its practice); in particular, general ones across particular topics of subject-matter.

Note: Theory of clinical research is subordinate to theory of clinical medicine [16] (just as, in epidemiological and clinical research, methods design is subordinate to objects design).

Translational research – Research aiming to transform a 'basic'-science discovery/concept into an innovation in the practice of medicine. (Example: 'drug development' up to regulatory approval of the drug's marketing.)

III – 3. TERMS AND CONCEPTS OF OBJECTS OF STUDY

Diagnostic probability function – See 'Gnostic probability function' (Notes 2 and 5-7).

Diagnostic test's properties – The two aspects of a test's diagnostic informativeness, constituting the objects of research on the test [16]:

1. *Post-test informativeness* – Given the post-test diagnostic profile, the extent to which the test result influences the (correct) diagnostic probability.

Note 1: If this were to be an object of study, at issue would be the *likelihood ratio* for each of the test results, contrasting illness present to illness absent, specific for each of the pre-test profiles. Given the generally very great multiplicity of these LRs, study of them is prohibitively impractical; but it is unnecessary besides.

Note 2: The diagnostician need not know how to move from the pre-test probability to the post-test probability, given that the test result has been obtained. In the face of this updated diagnostic profile, (s)he merely needs to know what the (correct) post-test probability is. And to this end, needed is research on the *post-test DPF*, for the domain of the decision node about the test's use. The test result has its degree of post-test informativeness represented in this function (along with those of the pre-test indicators), but this role is no concern of the diagnostician, given the availability of the test's result.

2. *Pre-test informativeness* – In the 'decision node' about the test's use, the probability that the test result would provide for transition from an 'inconclusive' pre-test probability to a 'conclusive' post-test probability.

Note 3: DPFs are needed for situations in which diagnostic probability-setting is needed; and these are situations in which a decision about an action – diagnostic testing, treatment, or referral – is to be taken. The presenting complaint prompts a defined aggregate of fact-findings from history and physical examination, leading to the profile for *clinical* diagnosis. This diagnosis – commonly quite 'inconclusive' – is prone to raise the question about invoking a particular test (possibly a composite of component tests); and for this decision needed is knowledge about the probability that the post-test diagnosis would be 'conclusive' – high or low enough for the decision about treatment or referral.

Note 4: For a study on a test's pre-test informativeness, a set of possibly 'conclusive' ranges of post-test probability needs to be defined (for the practitioner to

O. S. Miettinen, *Epidemiological Research: Terms and Concepts*,
DOI 10.1007/978-94-007-1171-6_10, © Springer Science+Business Media B.V. 2011

be able to focus on a chosen one, or pair, of these). For any given one of these, the object of study is the probability of a given range of post-test probability as a function of the pre-test indicators. (The dependent variate is an indicator of the range, the post-test DPFs realization falling in it.)

DPF – Diagnostic probability function.

Endpoint – See section III – 4.

EPF – Etiognostic probability function.

Etiognostic probability function – See 'Gnostic probability function' (Notes 3 and 5-7).

Explanatory trial* – See 'Explanatory versus pragmatic trial.'

Explanatory* versus pragmatic* trial – A duality in the purpose, and its corresponding intervention contrast, of a clinical trial.

   1. In an *explanatory* trial the object of study is the effect of a particular *agent* of intervention (typically a medication, or a surgical alteration of structure such as installment of a coronary artery bypass graft). The causal contrast thus is, conceptually, between the presence and the absence of the agent, but operationally it is between two treatments: treatment with the agent and treatment without the agent – between *verum* and *placebo/sham* treatment. Treatment with the agent is a practical necessity (for introduction of the agent to its recipient), while identical treatment without the agent – placebo/sham treatment, that is – is necessary for prevention of confounding by extraneous (non-agent) aspects of the treatment. An added reason for this pseudo-treatment can be the need for blinding the study.

   2. In a *pragmatic* trial the object of study is the effect of a particular *treatment*, without regard for what in the treatment produces the effect. The causal contrast thus is between this treatment (defined by an algorithm for the entire duration of follow-up) and an alternative for this – both of them candidates for being someone's treatment of choice. (The choice is for the recipient to make, whenever possible.)

Gnostic probability function – The generic object of quintessentially 'applied' clinical research [16].

   Note 1: Corresponding to the three genera of gnosis – diagnosis, etiognosis, and prognosis – the respective GPFs are *diagnostic* probability function (DPF), *etiognostic* probability function (EPF), and *prognostic* probability function (PPF).

   Note 2: A DPF addresses the probability – prevalence – of the illness at issue, in a particular domain of patient presentation (chief complaint, . . .), as a joint function of a set of diagnostic indicators (specifying the diagnostic profile, the union of the risk and manifestational subprofiles of this).

   Note 3: An EPF addresses the probability of causal/etiogenetic role for an antecedent (that was present in lieu of its defined alternative) for an illness (that is present), in a particular domain of the occurrence of the illness, as a joint function of a set of etiognostic indicators (specifying etiognostic profile, based on modifiers of the causal rate-ratio in the domain).

Note 4: A PPF may address, for a particular domain of prognostication, either the risk of a particular, still-absent illness developing; or it addresses the course of an already-existing illness – focusing on probability of sickness from the illness in the course of it, an outcome of the course, a complication of the illness, or an adverse effect of intervention on the course. With an outcome of the course of an illness a possible exception, the probability is a function of prognostic time; but it also is a function of the prognostic indicators at prognostic T_0 and the choice of intervention.

Note 5: A GPF is *scientific* if, and only if, it is rational in its (designed) form (for the domain at issue), and its content (of that form) derives from (gnostic) research.

Note 6: A scientific GPF can be, merely, the *result* of a gnostic study (original or derivative); but alternatively – and preferably – it expresses scientific *knowledge* (informed by gnostic research). GPFs of the latter type are the basis of (the practice of) truly scientific clinical medicine.

Note 7: A GPF is *quasi-scientific* if, and only if, it is scientific (rational) in form but its content represents experts' tacit knowledge without any input from gnostic research. (Cf. 'Gnostic expert paneling' in sect. III – 4.)

GPF – Gnostic probability function.

Intervention – See section I – 1. 2 and 'Outcomes research' (Note 2) in section III – 2.

Note: In the U. S. National Institutes of Health there has developed the pernicious habit of thinking about diagnostic testings as interventions [16]. (See 'Outcomes research' in sect. III – 2 and 'Screening' in sect. I – 1. 2.)

*Likelihood ratio** – See 'Diagnostic test's properties' (Note 1).

Link – Causal connection.

Note: The word, in this meaning, is commonly used by science reporters in the public media. It does not deserve to be used by researchers.

*Overparametrization/overfitting** – Concerning a regression model, the involvement of an excessive number of parameters in relation to the amount of information in the data.

Note 1: In logistic regression the here-relevant measure of the amount of information is $Np(1-p)$, where N is the number of datapoints and p is the proportion of these with $Y = 1$, and the measure of overparametrization is the number of parameters (Bs) in the model in proportion to $Np(1-p)$, this exceeding 0.05 or so.

Note 2: Given that the model (for a GPF) needs to be one with a rather large number of parameters, at issue here actually is *undersizing* of the study rather than overparametrization/overfitting of the model.

Note 3: The consequence of this undersizing is an unusual type of *bias*: relatively high values of the fitted function are biased upward, relatively low values being biased downward.

Note 4: Correction for the undersizing bias is termed *shrinkage*.

Placebo* – See 'Explanatory versus pragmatic trial.'

Post-test informativeness/probability – See 'Diagnostic test's properties.'

PPF – Prognostic probability function.

Pragmatic trial* – See 'Explanatory versus pragmatic trial.'

Pre-test informativeness/probability – See 'Diagnostic test's properties.'

Prognostic probability function – See 'Gnostic probability function' (Notes 4-7).

Receiver operating characteristic curve* – "A graphic means for assessing the ability of a screening or diagnostic test to discriminate between persons with and without the target disorder. For an ordinal or continuous diagnostic test, the ROC curve depicts the plot of all pairs of sensitivity and 1-specificity (false-positive probability) over all possible or chosen cutoff values" [4].

Note 1: A screening test is a diagnostic test, the initial one in pursuing diagnosis (rule-in) about a latent case of a particular illness.

Note 2: A diagnostic test's "ability to discriminate" – informativeness – is not a property of the test in isolation. It is a *marginal* property, conditional on the pre-test diagnostic profile. (Cf. 'Diagnostic test's properties.')

Note 3: Suitable measures of that informativeness are result-specific *likelihood ratios* conditional on the pre-test profile – insofar as such a multitude of parameters is considered relevant and practical to address. (Cf. 'Diagnostic test's properties.')

Note 4: For both the ROC and LR outlooks, a suitable *alternative* is needed. This alternative is study of the pre-test and post-test diagnostic probability functions and, also, the distribution of the test result conditionally on the pre-test profile. (See 'Diagnostic test's properties.')

ROC curve – Receiver operating characteristic curve.

III – 4. TERMS AND CONCEPTS OF METHODS OF STUDY

See note opening section II – 2.

Blinding* – In the methodology of a study, an arrangement making the observers unaware of certain facts (that might bias their observations); also: the counterpart of this in respect to the study subjects (notably as to the category of intervention to which they were assigned in an intervention-prognostic study, so as to prevent this influencing their engagement in extraneous interventions and/or their reporting on their experiences).

Note: If both the observers and subjects in a study are blinded, the study is said to be *double-blinded.*

Blocking* (synonym: restriction of randomization) – In the randomization of (allocations in) an experimental intervention-prognostic study (randomized trial), the feature of the randomization being performed separately within subsets – component 'blocks' – of the study subjects with the same allocation ratio(s) in all of these. (Cf. 'Randomization.')

Note: Blocking fully assures the balance (at T_0) in respect to the blocking factor, while randomization assures it only stochastically.

Clinical trial* (synonyms: randomized trial, randomized controlled trial) – An intervention-prognostic experiment for clinical medicine. See 'Randomized controlled trial.'

Note: The term is a bit of an euphemism, to avoid the unpleasant connotations commonly associated with 'experiment' when the subjects are humans. The term is a cognate of 'trying,' used in reference to intervention in clinical practice, free of any untoward connotations.

Cochrane collaboration* – "An international organization of clinicians, epidemiologists, patients, and others that aims to help health professional to make well-informed decisions about health care by preparing, maintaining, disseminating, and promoting the necessary systematic reviews of the effects of health care interventions. *Cochrane Reviews* are prepared and updated by collaborating authors working in a *Cochrane Collaborative Review Group* and using explicity defined methods to

O. S. Miettinen, *Epidemiological Research: Terms and Concepts*,
DOI 10.1007/978-94-007-1171-6_11, © Springer Science+Business Media B.V. 2011

minimize the effects of bias; where appropriate and feasible, meta-analysis is used to reduce imprecision" [4].

Complete randomization (antonym: restricted randomization) – Randomization of (allocations in) an experimental intervention-prognostic study (randomized trial) performed without any restriction by way of randomized blocks. See 'Randomization' (Note 1).

*Compliance** – A misnomer for a study subject's – study population member's – adherence to what (s)he presumably is committed to per 'informed consent.'

  Note: Compliance really means subordination/submission to an order. 'Compliance' in the meaning here should be replaced by 'adherence.'

Conclusion – See sections I – 2. 2 and II – 4.

*Confidence interval** – Misnomer for *imprecision* interval for a/the result of a study. (Cf. section II – 4.)

*Confounding by indication** – In an intervention study, confounding by the indication for the intervention (as is obvious from the term).

  Note 1: One of the major differences between etiogenetic and intervention studies, on the level of the object of study already, is that the former are generally about unintended effects, while the latter are mostly about *intended* effects [9]; and since the indication for intervention generally is an indication of the (prospective) outcome the risk of which is intended to be reduced by the intervention, the *indication is an inherent – ubiquitous – confounder* in the intervention versus no intervention contrast and a common possibility in inter-intervention contrasts as well [62, 63]. When the details of the indication are not subject to close documentation (for control of the confounding), the need is to *prevent* confounding by it – by resorting to experimentation with *randomization* as the basis for intervention allocation [62, 63].

  Note 2: Confounding by indication is commonly mistaken to be a form of selection bias (instead of confounding bias). But it is not bias of any form (in the study result); it is only a *potential source of confounding bias* – which confounding is to be prevented if it cannot be controlled.

  Note 3: Very distinct from confounding by indication is confounding by contra-indication [62, 63] – contra-indication generally being, if present at all, (1) very rare rather than ubiquitous, among the study subjects; (2) without inherent status as a determinant even of the unintended, rare outcomes that may be addressed (with generally quite wanting precision); and (3) generally quite readily subject to documentation.

  Note 4: Significantly, the I.E.A. dictionary [4] writes about confounding by indication with a reference only to the Editor himself, in 1998; and it is presented not as "a type of confounding" but of "confounding bias," and it is equated with bias from contra-indication, adding that "It shares some features with 'susceptibility bias,' 'procedure selection bias,' 'protopathic bias,' and 'selection bias.' "

Consent* – A person's agreement to submit to simulated care (diagnostic or interventive, in an experiment) and to the use of the data for research; or, to the use of the data on actual care for research.

Note 1: Ethics requires the consent to be *informed* – meaning well-informed, first as to the (true) implications, to the consenting person, of the consent relative to not consenting. An added meaning of well-informed consent is that the consenting person is made aware of the (true) motives for the solicitation of the consent (pecuniary, careerist, or whatever other self-serving motives first and foremost). For, a doctor is ethically bound to act in the best interest only of the client (as a matter of the unspoken 'fiducial contract' between them).

Note 2: *Equipoise** – "A state of genuine uncertainty about the genuine benefits or [*sic*] harms that may result from different exposures or interventions ... [it] is an indication for a randomized controlled trial" [4], meaning that it gives an ethical warrant for soliciting participation in an RCT. But the question is, Whose equipoise? the investigators'? The answer: For the solicitation, a first ethical requirement is that the potential participant be *compos mentis*, and that in the view of the relevant *scientific community* at large, there could be *potential study subjects* who, once (truly) well-informed and also compos mentis, would be willing to participate. And a well-informed person's decision to participate is not predicated on his/her equipoise. (S)he may wish to contribute to relevant research even with some perceived risk to his/her own health.

Note 3: In today's IRB-approved experiments (diagnostic or interventive) on human subjects, the solicitation of purportedly informed consent is, quite routinely, disingenuous. A telling indication of this is that, quite routinely, the information given out in the solicitation is intentionally kept unchanging throughout the period of subject accrual – deliberately excluding from it the evidence garnered in the study itself and, also, evidence from other simultaneously on-going similar studies.

Note 4: Apart from the requirement of obtaining informed consent, ethics of human experimentation is now taken to involve the work of a *Data Safety and Monitoring Board*, "charged with assessing the progress of clinical trials and to recommend whether the trial should continue, be modified, or be discontinued. More specifically, the DSMB approves the protocol, ... ; and DSMBs review interim analyses ... performed prior to study completion" [64].

Note 5: If the trial participants were (truly) well-informed, not only at enrolment but in the course of their trial participations also, there would be *no need, nor justification, for DSMBs* to take decisions about trials' continuations/stoppings. The participants would, individually, take the decisions; and stoppings by DSMB decisions would thus be replaced by vanishing of the continually participating volunteers.

Note 6: Even though the language here focuses on trials in clinical research, epidemiologists in their research for community medicine also engage in trials with individuals as the units of observation. Examples: trials on screening for a cancer, trials on chemoprevention of cancer, and trials on vaccinations – recently including vaccination in the prevention of cervical cancer.

Note 7: While an individual's enrolment into participation in a health-related study – non-experimental study included – is generally supposed to require, as a matter of ethics, the individual's informed consent, in many jurisdictions cancer patients are legally obligated to provide data for cancer research (by cancer registries). Operative in this can be said to be not *deontological* but *teleological* – utilitarian – ethics, the creed which, in the words of J. S. Mill, "accepts as the foundation of morality, Utility of the Greatest Happiness of People" [65]. Deontological (duty-based) ethics is supposed to be the sole concern in clinical research, but a more natural ethical stance in community research can be seen to be the teleological (goals-oriented) one, though with due respect for individual values (re personal happiness).

*Contamination** – In a randomized trial, non-adherence to the assigned category of intervention in the form of crossing over to an/the other category (irrespective of whether at issue is the study subject's or the investigators' non-adherence to the trial's protocol).

Note 1: 'Contamination' in reference to protocol non-adherence is as ugly a term as is 'discharge' for the termination of hospitalization.

Note 2: There really is no genuine need for a term specific to intervention crossover as a particular subtype of protocol non-adherence in an intervention trial, one that distinguishes this from other, equally deleterious types of non-adherence to the intervention protocol.

*Control** – See 'Randomized controlled trial' (Note 2).

Data Safety and Monitoring Board – See 'Consent' (Note 4).

Diagnostic study – The structure ('architecture') dictated by logic for any study intended to serve advancement of the (scientific) knowledge-base of diagnostication (i.e., of setting diagnostic probability for the presence of the illness at issue). Its elements are: (1) study base constituted by a series of person-moments from the domain of diagnosis (chief complaint, . . .); and (2) for the study base, documented counterpart of the (designed) object of study (diagnostic probability function – logistic).

Note 1: Always to be reported is the result without shrinkage; but the result with shrinkage also needs to be derived and reported whenever at issue is the first study (original or derivative) on the object function and the result might be applied as such (without its translation to knowledge; cf. 'Gnostic expert paneling').

Note 2: A diagnostic study, in this sense, may address a test's informativeness in the sense of producing both a pre-test and a post-test DPF, thereby providing for studying the test's *informativeness* (see 'Diagnostic test's properties' in sect. III – 3). In such a study, a measure of this could be $I = 1 - R^2$, R being the 'coefficient' of correlation between the pre- and post-test probabilities. ($R^2 = 1$ means $I = 0$, complete uninformativeness of the test result.)

Note 3: Study of a test's *informativeness* preferably has a different object of study, one not focusing on DPFs. The dependent variate does not signify the presence/absence of the illness but, instead, whether the post-test probability falls in a particular range; and the object of (each component) study is the probability of this as a function of the pre-test indicators. (See 'Diagnostic test's properties,' Notes 3 and 4, in sect. III – 3.)

*Double blinding** – See 'Blinding' (Note).

Endpoint – In a prognostic study (RCT, say), the point at which follow-up ends on account of the outcome event occurring.

*Equipoise** – See 'Consent' (Note 2).

*Ethics** – See 'Consent' (Note 7) and 'Institutional Review Board' (Note 1).

Etiognostic study – The structure ('architecture') dictated by logic for any study of etiogenesis, intended to serve advancement of the (scientific) knowledge-base of etiognostication (i.e., of setting probability for causal – etiogenetic – role for an antecedent of an illness). The structure is the general one of an etiologic/etiogenetic study. (Special is only the stage of the evolution of the knowledge – in which quantification has come to follow hypothesis-testing – and the richness of detail in the occurrence relation needed for clinical etiognosis.)

Expert – A gnostician who, in dealing with cases from the domain at issue, is judged (by colleagues) to be as competent as anyone.
   Note 1: At present, an expert's competence in setting gnostic probabilities is, quite exclusively, a matter of *tacit* knowledge in particular cases that come up – knowledge accrued largely on the basis of *personal experience* with cases from the presentation domain at issue. It thus is not knowledge derived – collectively – from quintessentially applied clinical research (via gnostic expert paneling).
   Note 2: In the now-foreseeable future, it will be generally understood that (1) the knowledge-base of clinical medicine can be – and needs to be – codified in the form of gnostic probability functions; and that (2) quasi-scientific GPFs, representing experts' tacit knowledge without inputs from research on the GPFs, can be developed quite rapidly and inexpensively, without having to await the results of (the still essentially non-existent) research on GPFs. Given this understanding – and the ever-mounting pressures of quality-assurance and cost-containment – clinical gnosticians in general will, in the foreseeable future already, function like experts typically do, their practices guided by *gnostic expert systems* [16].
   Note 3: As research on GPFs gets underway in earnest, true understanding of such research becomes an important added element in the competence of expert gnosticians in the various disciplines ('specialties') of clinical medicine.

Gnostic expert paneling – Translation of evidence into practice-guiding knowledge about a gnostic probability function: A panel of experts (on the gnosis at issue) are presented with vignettes (scores of them) of hypothetical patients, each profile supplemented by the value implied by the relevant study result (if available); the panel members specify, independently, their perception of the gnostic probability in each of the (hypothetical) cases, and the median of these probabilities is derived for each case; these medians are translated into the corresponding GPF by fitting it to the data, both without and with shrinkage [16].

*Goodness of fit** – Concerning the result of regression 'analysis,' the extent to which the observed means of the dependent variate conform to the respective 'estimates' from the empirical (fitted) regression function across various ranges of the 'estimates' (in a diagnostic study, say.)

*Hawthorne effect** – In experiments on human subjects (RCTs, say), the study subjects' changes of behavior not intended by the investigators yet consequential to the study outcome(s).

   Note: The effect fundamentally is that of increased health-consciousness, and its consequent changes of behavior generally are intended to change the course of health for the better (by actions that are extraneous from the vantage of the experiment). To the extent that the Hawthorne effect is there in a consequential way, the prognostic results of RCTs conditional on the choice of intervention tend to have a bias toward more favorable outcome(s).

Hierarchy of evidence – See section II – 4.

*Informed consent** – See 'Consent' (Note 1).

*Institutional Review Board** – In the U. S., the committee each research institution is required to have for evaluation of each plan, in the institution, for a study that would involve human subjects. The IRB is to pass judgment about whether the study would be ethical and, in this sense, admissible.

   Note 1: For a study involving human subjects to be ethically admissible, it is to satisfy the imperatives of both teleological and deontological ethics. *Teleologically*, the study – like any other action/activity of humans – is (to be intended) to enhance the aggregate happiness of mankind (i.e., to have utility – positive – from this 'mass' perspective); and *deontologically*, it must not impose on the study subjects any disutility (suffering or deprivation) that teleologically is uncalled for and/or is unacceptable to the study subjects – compos mentis and, in relevant respects, fully informed. (Gr. *teleos*, 'complete, final'; Gr. *deon*, 'binding, needful.')

   Note 2: An IRB – this 'ethical' committee – acts unethically if it approves a study without full assurance – full knowledge – that the study actually is ethically admissible; and an IRB makes this ethical error most generally and most fundamentally by presuming to be qualified to pass ethical judgments on whatever study involving human subjects. For, such a study is unethical – an unethical imposition on the study subjects – if it is wanting in quality-optimization of its object(s) and/or methods designs, including in maximization of the study's efficiency; and it is unethical if the 'informed consent' is sought without making the study subjects truly fully-informed. See 'Consent.'

Note 3: The elements in this quality-optimization in this information-transmission are matters of extra-ethical expertise and inter-institutional in nature; and thus, the only justifiable, truly ethical role for an IRB really is making sure that genuine expertise on these matters has been brought to bear on, and heeded, in the design of the study and of the consent form. For intra-institutionally, horrendous contraventions of research ethics can take place, even in ostensibly legitimate institutions, starting from the studies' object(s) designs [66]. And an IRB, however well-intentioned, generally is not qualified to judge the adequacy of the information input into the solicitation of informed consent for study participation – to act on behalf of the relevant scientific community in this judgment. (Cf. 'Consent.')

*Intention to treat** – In the result of an RCT, the quality that its referent is the contrast formed by the randomizations, regardless of whether the interventions actually conformed to the randomized assignments.

Note: The ITT quality of an RCT result implies freedom from confounding (systematic) at T_0 of prognostic time; but it implies bias on account of incompleteness (if any) of adherence to the randomly assigned interventions.

Intervention-prognostic study (synonym: intervention study) – See 'Intervention study.'

*Intervention study** (synonym: intervention-prognostic study) – The structure ('architecture') dictated by logic for any study on the intended effect(s) of an intervention. Its elements are: (1) the study base constituted by a segment (early) of the prospective course of a cohort, with subcohorts according to the contrasted interventions, this divergence prevailing as of cohort T_0 (but not before); and (2) for the study base, documented counterpart of the designed object of study.

Note 1: At present in RCTs, as for the implicit object of study, the effect of an intervention (relative to its alternative) is commonly addressed in terms of deriving from the data the 'hazard ratio' – meaning the empirical value of this parameter – together with the 95% 'confidence interval' to go with this. But, bringing the structure of the etiologic study (sect. II – 4) suitably to bear, an (empirical) prognostic probability function (of prognostic time, intervention, and prognostic indicators at cohort/prognostic T_0) can, and should, be derived from the data [9, 16] – upon suitable design of the form of this (in the study's object design). Rather than a mere intervention study, such a study is an *intervention-prognostic study*.

Note 2: While the structure of an intervention study has that of the RCT as its paradigm, an intervention study need not be experimental, to have experimental arrangement of the contrasted treatments. The structure can be *quasi-experimental* in its genesis (see sect. I – 2. 2).

Note 3: See also 'Prognostic study.'

IRB – Institutional Review Board.

Kaplan-Meier-Greenwood statistics* – The Kaplan-Meier 'point estimate' together with the Greenwood standard error for the complement of cumulative incidence in the time-course of a cohort (with terminations of follow-up also for reasons other than the event at issue).

Note 1: When at issue is *survival* in a cohort of patients diagnosed with a particular illness (cancer, notably), the K-M 'estimate' represents the cohort's rate of surviving the illness at issue for a given period of time since cohort T_0 in the absence of deaths from other causes – that is, when (counterfactually) regarding the illness at issue as the only cause of death.

Note 2: The *K-M survival rate* [67] is derived by focusing, in the cohort's follow-up time, on the points at which deaths from the cause/illness at issue occur. When the first (known) death from this cause occurred, the number of survivors under follow-up changed from S_1 to $S_1 - 1$, and the survival rate became $(S_1 - 1)/S_1$. If, in the follow-up period at issue, a total of d deaths from the cause at issue occurred, the K-M survival rate was the product of d proportions of this type:

$$R = \prod_1^d (S_i - 1)/S_i (i = 1, \ldots, d).$$

This rate is, thus, derived without any regard for the numbers of losses to follow-up as well as of deaths from other causes in the time period at issue, including in the subperiod of time after the last death from the cause at issue (in which period the size of the subcohort still under follow-up may have declined to however meaningless a number).

Note 3: The Greenwood standard error for the K-M survival rate (R) is [69]

$$SE = R \left[\sum_1^d 1/S_i(S_i - 1) \right]^{1/2}.$$

Involved in this is ML estimation of the binomial variances. Based on the corresponding unbiased estimates, the counterpart of this is [68]

$$SE = R \left[\sum_1^d 1/(S_i - 1)^2 \right]^{1/2}.$$

(In general, unbiased 'estimates' are used and preferred. This tends to be forgotten in the context of the readily obtained ML values for the Bernoulli and binomial variances.)

Note 4: The complement of the K-M survival rate a modern epidemiologist naturally thinks of as the *cumulative incidence-rate* of death from the illness at issue in the time period at issue. Like the K-M survival rate, this CIR is conditional on not succumbing to a 'competing' cause of death (as it is based on incidence density of the death at issue, inherently among survivors). Specifically, with the survival period divided into a set of subperiods, and with d_j deaths from the cause at issue occurring in the jth subperiod of duration t_j and population-time T_j of follow-up, the complement of the K-M survival rate can be derived as [69]

$$CIR = 1 - exp\left[\sum_j (d_j/T_j)t_j\right].$$

This generally is in close agreement with the K-M survival rate.

Note 5: The SE relevant to this CIR is that of the time-integral of incidence density (in the exponential). This is:

$$SE = \left[\sum_j d_j(t_j/T_j)^2\right]^{1/2}.$$

With this SE applied to the exponent in the CIR, 'confidence' limits for the theoretical CIR are, generally, in close accord with the complements of the K-M-G limits.

Note 6: SE-based limits are not first-principles limits. In the case at issue here, they are not, even, inherently bound to remain within the 0-to-1 range. The CIR approach, however, lends itself to derivation of first-principles limits, and not only asymptotic limits (like these SE-based ones) but 'exact' ones as well [69].

Note 7: An eminent alternative to the K-M survival rate is the *Nelson-Aalen* 'estimator,'

$$R = \sum_1^d 1/S_i;$$

but preferable to this can be taken to be [69]

$$R = \sum_1^d 1/(S_i - 1/2).$$

Likelihood – A misnomer in reference to a study result when saying that one group had a higher, or lower, 'likelihood' of the outcome when at issue is merely an empirical difference between two rates. (Cf. 'Result' in sect. II – 4.)

Meta-analysis* – In a derivative study, synthesis of the results of original studies.

Note: The term is a misnomer. For one, the 'analysis' actually is synthesis (cf. 'Analysis and synthesis' in sect. I – 2. 2). For another, at issue still is 'analysis,' rather than something that transcends it. (Cf. 'meta-physics.')

Overparametrization/overfitting* – See section III – 3.

Prognostic study – The structure ('architecture') dictated by logic for any study of the course of health, intended to serve advancement of the (scientific) knowledge base of prognostication. Its elements are: (1) study population constituted by a cohort whose members are enrolled from the domain of the prognostication; (2) study base constituted by the study cohort's prospective course (in cohort and prognostic time); and (3) for the study base, the documented counterpart of the (designed) object of study (prognostic probability function).

Note 1: The prime generic example of a prognostic study is the *randomized controlled trial* (of interventions) addressing a prognostic probability function.

Note 2: For documentation of a PPF for a *state* of health, contributions to the study base are not terminated by 'endpoint' events. A sample – in principle any type of outcome-independent sample (finite) – of the (infinite number of) person-moments of the study base is selected and documented, and the PPF is fitted to these data – without and with shrinkage. The state of health at a given time may be the then frequency of episodes of sickness from the illness (epilepsy, say) – the then moving average of this frequency.

Note 3: For documentation of a PPF for an *event* of health, contributions to the study base are terminated by the event's occurrence. Regarding the event, the case series is identified and documented in respect to intervention history (type of intervention and time since cohort/prognostic T_0) and prognostic profile at T_0. The case series is supplemented by a base series, selected as a *representative* (simple random) sample of the study base and documented analogously with the case series. The logistic counterpart of the log-linear model for the event's incidence density (as a function of prognostic time, choice of intervention, and prognostic indicators) is fitted to the data on these two series. The result for the event's incidence density is the fitted logistic function's exponential multiplied by b / B, where b is the size of the base series and B is the amount of population-time constituting the study base. The integral of this function over prognostic time is translated into its corresponding cumulative incidence and, thereby, to the result for the prognostic probability function [9].

*Randomization** – Random assignment/allocation of study subjects to particular ones of the compared/contrasted interventions.

Note 1: In *complete* randomization, all of the allocations are mutually independent, except for the possible role of a preset allocation ratio.

Note 2: In *restricted* randomization, a given allocation ratio is designed to be the result of randomization within defined 'blocks' of study subjects (patients from a particular participating clinic, say), but among the blocks the randomizations are mutually independent.

*Randomized controlled trial** (synonyms: randomized trial, clinical trial) – An experimental intervention-study, one in which the allocations to the contrasted interventions are based on randomization.

Note 1: An RCT is usually a *parallel* trial, one with treatment-specific subcohorts formed and then followed in parallel in calendar time. But an alternative to this is a *cross-over trial*, in which the study subjects change from one of the contrasted treatments to the other one in the course of their follow-up. This type of trial, too, can be randomized, now in defining the individual sequences in the use of the contrasted interventions.

Note 2: The meaning of '*control*' in this context is not that there is experimental control of the allocations to the contrasted interventions; this is the meaning of 'trial' (i.e., 'experiment'). Instead, the meaning is this: In studying the effect(s) of a particular intervention, experience with a cohort subjected to this intervention shows only what happens with this intervention; the experience does not show what would have happened without this intervention. To learn about the latter, a 'control' cohort subjected to the intervention's alternative is included in the trial.

Note 3: The term *'trial'* in this context is a bit of an euphemism (cf. Note under 'Clinical trial'). And once a trial is *randomized*, it inherently also is controlled (in the meaning of Note 2 above), so that *'randomized trial'* should be preferred over 'randomized controlled trial' as the term for this type of clinical study.

Randomized trial (synonyms: randomized controlled trial, clinical trial) – See 'Randomized controlled trial' (Note 3).

RCT – Randomized controlled trial.

RCTism – The doctrinary outlook in terms of which even diagnostic testing is intervention (on the course of health), intended to have efficacy/effectiveness, and thus is to be assessed by means of RCTs. (Cf. 'Outcomes research' in sect. III – 2.)

Reduction – A misnomer for a result consistent with a reducing effect.

Note: The word derives from a transitive verb. It has to do with causation (a noumenon) which the difference or ratio does not inherently represent.

Regression toward the mean * – The tendency of a repeat observation (with chance error) to be closer to the mean.

Replication * – Concerning a measurement, its repetition with a view to reduction of chance error in the result; also: concerning an object of study, conducting a new study on it with the essentials of design and protocol as in a previous study on it – though in a different place at a different time and, generally, with a different precision (on account of different efficiency and/or size) – with a view to potential corroboration. (Cf. sect. I – 2. 2.)

Restricted randomization – See 'Randomization' (Note 2).

Sample size determination * – See section II – 4.

Note: 'Sample size determination' is outstanding among the negative contributions of statistics to statistical science. The most common statistical consultation for study design by clinicians concerns 'sample size determination.'

Shrinkage * – In the context of 'overparametrization' of a regression model and its consequent 'overfitting' of the model (sect. III – 3), correction for the bias in the 'estimates' for the dependent parameter, resulting from the large number of parameters in the model in proportion to the number of units of observation in the study.

Note 1: 'Overparametrization' is a misnomer in this context, and so also is 'overfitting.' 'Overparametrization' properly refers to a flaw in object design, for a diagnostic study in particular, and this is not what actually is at issue here. The context of the diagnostic probability-setting is prone to involve dozens of diagnostic indicators, and a reasonable regression model even more independent parameters; and a biased result from the fitting of the model is not really a result of a flaw in the parametrization of the model nor in its fitting to the study data. The bias actually is a consequence of *undersizing* of the study – insufficient number of units of observation in proportion to the number of parameters in the model. (Cf. sect. III – 3.)

Note 2: The nature of the bias is unusual, given that the 'estimates' for the dependent parameter from the fitted 'polymultiple' regression have no systematic error in the usual, across-the-board meaning. Instead, the resulting relatively low 'estimates' involve a downward bias, the relatively high ones an upward bias. This result-specific bias arises from the fact that, in the database, the relatively low values of the dependent variate are prone to involve a negative 'error' (chance element), the relatively high values a positive one – and the fitting of the polymultiple regression model traces these patterns of chance in addition to reflecting the actual values of the parameters in the model.

Note 3: This extraordinary type of bias – a feature not of the fitted coefficients but of the linear compound of these, when viewed as the empirical value of the dependent parameter conditional on the (polymultiple) set of independent variates – has the extraordinary character that it is reduced – and ultimately eliminated – by increasing size of the database, as in moving from an original study to a derivative study drawing from several original studies. Thus, correction for the bias – shrinkage, that is – is called for only insofar as the result, whether from the first original study or a subsequent derivative study, will be applied as such – before bias-reduction from further contributions to the aggregate of evidence (about the magnitudes of the model's independent parameters).

Note 4: Among the various available ways of effecting the requisite shrinkage, the most intuitive one arguably is the '*leave-out-one*' method: Of the N datapoints, one is left out in fitting the model (to the other $N-1$), and this fitted model is used to derive the value $\hat{Y}_1$ corresponding to the left-out value Y_1. This process is repeated for each of the other datapoints, leading to data pairs $(Y_i, \hat{Y}_i), i = 1, 2, \ldots, N$. In the usual context of the regression model being logistic, the next phase is to fit a univariate regression model for the mean of the logit of Y, involving $B_0 + B_1 X$, where X is the logit of the 'estimate' based on the fitting without shrinkage. In this, the need for shrinkage is manifest in $\hat{B}_1 < 1$. Finally, then, the result with the requisite shrinkage is, for the logit of the mean (*P*) of Y, incorporated in $\hat{B}_0 + \hat{B}_1 L$, where L is the linear compound from the initial fitting – 'overfitting' of the polymultiple regression model (requiring shrinkage by the factor $\hat{B}_1$).

*Survival analysis** – See 'Kaplan-Meier-Greenwood statistics.'

*Systematic review** – A review of and report on all original studies on the object at issue, especially if 'meta-analysis' is involved.

REFERENCES

1. McCall RJ. Basic Logic. Second edition. New York: Barnes & Noble, Inc., 1952; p. 1 ff.
2. Moore FE. Committee on design and analysis of studies. Am J Publ Health 1960; 50: 10–9.
3. MacMahon B, Pugh TF, Ipsen J. Epidemiologic Methods. Boston: Little, Brown and Company, 1960.
4. Porta M (Editor), Greenland S, Last JM (Associate Editors). A Dictionary of Epidemiology. Fifth edition. Oxford: Oxford University Press, 2008.
5. Miettinen OS. Theoretical developments. In: Holland WW, Olsen J, Florey C du V (Editors). The Development of Modern Epidemiology. Personal Reports by Those Who Were There. Oxford: Oxford University Press, 2007.
6. Miettinen OS. Book review. M. Porta (Editor), S. Greenland & J. M. Last (Associate editors). A Dictionary of Epidemiology. A Handbook Sponsored by the I.E.A. Eur J Epidemiol 2008; 23: 813–7.
7. Miettinen OS. Etiologic research: needed revisions of concepts and principles. Scand J Work, Envir & Health 1999: 6 (special issue): 484–90.
8. Miettinen OS, Flegel KM. Elementary concepts of medicine: VI. Genesis of illness: pathogenesis, aetiogenesis. J Eval Clin Pract 2003; 9: 325–7.
9. Miettinen OS. Etiologic study vis-à-vis intervention study. Eur J Epidemiol 2010; 25: 671–5.
10. Miettinen OS, Flegel KM. Elementary concepts of medicine: III. Illness: somatic anomaly with ... J Eval Clin Pract 2003; 315–7.
11. Miettinen OS, Flegel KM. Elementary concepts of medicine: V. Disease: one of the main subtypes of illness. J Eval Clin Pract 2003; 9: 321–3.
12. Miettinen OS. Theoretical Epidemiology. Principles of Occurrence Research in Medicine. New York: John Wiley & Sons, 1985.
13. Bacon F. The Essays or Counsels Civil and Moral. Oxford: Oxford University Press, 1999; p. 134.
14. Berlin I. The Proper Study of Mankind. An Anthology of Essays (Hardy H, Hausheer R, Editors). London: Chatto & Windus, 1990; p. 61.
15. Miettinen OS. Ignoring critique, attacking the critic. Eur J Epidemiol 2010; 25; 149.
16. Miettinen OS. Up from Clinical Epidemiology & EBM. Dordrecht: Springer, 2011.
17. Miettinen OS. Important concepts in epidemiology. In: Olsen J, Saracci R, Trichopoulos D (Editors). Teaching Epidemiology. Third Edition. Oxford: Oxford University Press, 2010.
18. Marti-Ibañez F [Editor]. The Epic of Medicine. New York: Clarkson N. Potter, Inc., 1962; p. xi.
19. Miettinen OS. The modern scientific physician: 2. Medical science versus scientific medicine. CMAJ 2001; 165: 591–2.
20. Miettinen OS, Flegel KM. Elementary concepts of medicine: I. Medicine: challenges with its concepts. J Eval Clin Pract 2003; 9: 307–9.
21. Miettinen OS. The modern scientific physician: 1. Can practice be science? CMAJ 2001; 165: 441–2.

22. Wertz G. Divide and Conquer. A Comparative History of Medical Specialization. Oxford: Oxford University Press, 2006.
23. Steurer J, Bachmann LM, Miettinen OS. Etiology in a taxonomy of illnesses. Eur J Epidemiol 2006; 21: 85–9.
24. Miettinen OS. Proportion of disease caused or prevented by a given exposure, trait or intervention. Am J Epidemiol 1974; 99: 325–32.
25. Miettinen OS. Evidence in medicine: invited commentary. CMAJ 1998; 158: 215–21.
26. Evidence-Based Medicine Working Group. Evidence-based medicine. A new approach to teaching the practice of medicine. JAMA 1992; 268: 2420–5.
27. Sackett DL, Straus SE, Richardson WS, et alii. Evidence-Based Medicine. How to Practice and Teach EBM. Second edition. Edinburgh: Churchill Livingstone, 2000.
28. Miettinen OS, Caro JJ. Foundations of medical diagnosis: What actually are the parameters involved in Bayes' theorem? Statist Med 1994; 13: 201–9.
29. Miettinen OS, Flegel KM. Elementary concepts of medicine: IV. Sickness from illness and in health. J Eval Clin Pract 2003; 9: 319–20.
30. Sargent R-M. Analysis and synthesis. In: Heilbron JL (Editor). The Oxford Companion to the History of Modern Science. Oxford: Oxford University Press, 2003.
31. Kant I. Critique of Pure Reason (translated by Meiklejohn JMD). Amherst (NY): Prometheus Books, 1990; p. 7.
32. Sargent R-M. Causality. In: Heilbron JL (Editor in Chief). The Oxford Companion to the History of Modern Science. Oxford: Oxford University Press, 2003.
33. Miettinen OS. Screening for a cancer: the pundits at a crossroads. Manuscript, to be published.
34. Rosenberg A. Philosophy of Science. A Contemporary Introduction. Second edition. New York: Routledge, 2000; pp. 22, 89.
35. Laudan R. Observation and experiment. In: Heilbron JL (Editor). The Oxford Companion to the History of Modern Science. Oxford: Oxford University Press, 2003.
36. Olesko K. Precision and accuracy. In: Heilbron JL (Editor). The Oxford Companion to the History of Modern Science. Oxford: Oxford University Press, 2003.
37. Laudan R. Proof. In: Heilbron JL (Editor in Chief). The Oxford Companion to the History of Modern Science. Oxford: Oxford University Press, 2003.
38. von Mises L. Human Action. A Treatise in Economics. Third, revised edition. Chicago: Contemporary Books, Inc., 1966; p. 10.
39. Pielke RA. The Honest Broker. Making Sense of Science in Policy and Politics. Cambridge: Cambridge University Press, 2007; p. v (in a quote from Lord May).
40. Liberati A, Chatziandreau E, Miettinen OS. Health care research: What is it about? Quality Assurance in Health Care 1989; 1: 249–57.
41. Hill AB. The environment and disease: association or causation. Proc R Soc Med 1965; 58: 295–300.
42. Proctor RN. The Nazi War on Cancer. Princeton: Princeton University Press, 1999.
43. Miettinen OS. Screening for a cancer: a sad chapter in today's epidemiology. Eur J Epidemiol 2008; 23: 647–53.
44. Miettinen OS. Screening for a cancer: thinking before rethinking. Eur J Epidemiol 2010; 25: in press.
45. Miettinen OS. Stratification by a multivariate confounder score. Am J Epidemiol 1976; 104: 609–20.
46. Miettinen OS. Estimability and estimation in case-referent studies. Am J Epidemiol 1976; 103: 226–35.
47. Stang A, Poole C, Kuss O. The ongoing tyranny of statistical significance testing in biomedical research. Eur J Epidemiol 2010; 25: 225–30.
48. Rothman KJ. Curbing type I and type II errors. Eur J Epidemiol 2010; 25: 223–4.
49. Ziliak ST, McCloskey DN. The Cult of Statistical Significance. How the Standard Error Costs Us Jobs, Justice, and Lives. Ann Arbor: The University of Michigan Press, 2008; pp. 2, 5.
50. Fletcher RH, Fletcher SN. Clinical Epidemiology. The Essentials. Fourth edition. Philadelphia: Lippincott Williams & Wilkins, 2005; pp. 2–3.

51. Hulley SB et alii. Designing Clinical Research. Third edition. Philadelphia: Lippincott Williams & Wilkins, 2007; p. xiii.
52. Glasser SP (Editor). Essentials of Clinical Research. Dordrecht: Springer, 2008; p. 4.
53. Grobbee DE, Hoes AW. Clinical Epidemiology. Principles, Methods, and Applications for Clinical Research. Boston: Jones and Bartlett Publishers, 2008; p. xi.
54. Cochrane AL. Effectiveness and Efficiency. Random Reflections on Health Services. London: Nuttfield Provincial Hospitals Trust, 1972; p. 2.
55. U. S. Congress, Office of Technology Assessment. Assessing the Efficacy of Medical Technologies. OTA – H – 75. Washington, DC: U. S. Government Printing Office, 1975.
56. U. S. Congress, Office of Technology Assessment. Identifying Health Technologies That Work. Washington, DC: U. S. Government Printing Office, 1994.
57. Thornbury JR. Why should radiologists be interested in technology assessment and outcomes research? Am J Radiol 1994; 163: 1027–30.
58. Hillman B. Outcomes research and cost-effectiveness analysis for diagnostic imaging research. Editorial. Radiol 1994; 193: 307–10.
59. Hillman BJ, Gatsonis C, Sullivan DC. American College of Radiology Imaging Network: new national cooperative group for conducting clinical trials of medical imaging technologies. Radiol 1999; 213: 641–5.
60. Epstein A. The outcomes movement – will it take us where we want to go? NEJM 1990; 323: 266–70.
61. Gold MR, Siegel JE, Russell LB, Weinstein MC (Editors). Cost-effectiveness in Health and Medicine. New York: Oxford University Press, 1996.
62. Miettinen OS. Efficacy of therapeutic practice: will epidemiology provide the answers? In: Melmon KL (Editor). Drug Therapeutics. Concepts for Physicians. New York: Elsevier – North Holland, 1980.
63. Miettinen OS. The need for randomization in the study of intended effects. Statist Med 1983; 2: 267–71.
64. Glasser SP, Williams OD. Data Safety and Monitoring Boards (DSMBs). In: Glasser SB (Editor). Essentials of Clinical Research. Dordrecht (NL): Springer, 2008.
65. Wiggins D. Ethics. Twelve Lectures on the Philosophy of Morality. London: Penquin Books, 2006; p. 147.
66. Scull A. Madhouse. A Tragic Tale of Megalomania and Modern Medicine. New Haven: Yale University Press, 2008.
67. Kaplan EL, Meier P. Nonparametric estimation from incomplete observations. J Am Stat Assoc 1958; 53: 457–81.
68. Greenwood M. A report on the natural duration of cancer. In: Reports on Public Health and Medical Subjects, Vol 33. London: His Majesty's Stationery Office, 1926; pp. 1–26.
69. Miettinen OS. Survival analysis: up from Kaplan-Meier-Greenwood. Eur J Epidemiol 2008; 23: 585–92.

INDEX

Listed below are, in their alphabetical order, all of the terms in sections I – 1. 2, I – 2. 2, I – 3. 2, II – 2-4, III – 2-4, and III – 2-4. Associated with each term is specification of the section(s) in which the term appears.

HIERARCHY OF CONCEPTS

What follows is my suggestion for the sequence in which concepts might best (most logically) be introduced (and justified) – for their most ready apprehension by the students – in an *introductory course* on epidemiological research (cf. Introduction in this book).

The sequence (and coverage) I here suggest is predicated on two *premises*:

1. Each student is preparing – or considering preparation – for a career in 'epidemiological' research – the actual meaning of 'epidemiological' possibly being that of 'meta-epidemiological clinical.'
2. Each student is suitably prepared for the course: (S)he has studied the here-relevant statistics (sect. I – 3), or (s)he is taking a course on those concepts parallel with this one; and (s)he has a sufficient level of proficiency in English (the lingua franca of modern science and, hence, the language of this course).

The point of departure in this course naturally is to be the concept of *epidemiology*, with the understanding that this is the segment of medicine that concerns morbidity in the community/population an epidemiologist is caring for, morbidity in its components specific to particular illnesses, these illness-specific morbidities in terms of rates of the occurrence of the respective illnesses. Grasping the full burden of this statement requires possession of a number of concepts other than that of epidemiology, from the concept of medicine to those of *rate*, starting from rate per se and then introducing the duality constituted by rates of incidence and those of prevalence. This will naturally lead to the concepts of adjustment and standardization of rates.

Where a clinician's concern is to prevent a case of an illness from occurring in an individual, an epidemiologist's corresponding concern is to reduce *morbidity* from the illness, by community-level preventive measures. While all of community medicine is *preventive medicine*, there now is considerable confusion among academic epidemiologists about the scope of preventive medicine, as viewed from the vantage of epidemiology. The course should develop a tenable concept of preventive medicine, in part because this term remains in use as a synonym for 'epidemiology' and 'community medicine' (along with 'social medicine').

The conception of epidemiology as community-level preventive medicine is made more concrete by coming to appreciate the principal *modalities* of preventive care in community medicine: education, regulation, and service. More to the same effect is delineation of what, in generic terms, tends to be involved in each of these three. A point of particular note that thus arises is that an epidemiologist's health-education pertaining to prevention of a particular illness is mass education of the individuals in the community, about self-care, with the content the same as in the corresponding aggregate of education/teaching/counseling in clinical preventive care. The mass education needs to involve the distinction-making that is inherent in the preventive care by clinicians. Individuals in the population need to be guided to the appropriate source (website) for guidance as to risk assessment, etc.

Such understanding of the nature of the practice of community medicine implies the nature of its *knowledge-base*: The proximal aim of the practice typically is removal of health hazards, behavioral and environmental (micro- and macro-environmental); only exceptionally is it invocation of an intervention (a vaccination, most notably, for constitutional change). The knowledge-base thus is about health hazards – their health effects – first and foremost; and to a minor extent it is about the effects of preventive interventions.

The knowledge-base of community-level preventive medicine in respect to health hazards is about causal origin – etiology, *etiogenesis* – of illness. The students need to achieve a secure grasp of the concept of etiogenesis of illness, this pari passu with the concept of pathogenesis. They need to learn that at issue in this is one of the two fundamental types of cause-effect relation that are of concern in medicine; and they need to learn to distinguish it, securely, from the other one, which mainly has to do with intended effects of interventions, preventive and other.

The topic of the knowledge-base of epidemiology (its practice) leads to the concept of science and that of *research* in it, original and derivative, including the concept of evidence as the product of a piece of research, a study. The students get to understand that epidemiological research does not constitute a science; and that scientific knowledge is not the direct product of epidemiological research. They also get to appreciate that some epidemiological studies (on rates) are not pieces of research but, instead, matters of particularistic fact-finding.

Now the students are ready to be introduced to the concept of etio-logic/*etiogenetic study*. In this, the natural beginning is the intuitive understanding that of central importance in this is a *case series* of the illness – successively identified cases documented in respect to the risk factor at issue.

It is good to think about this case series first on the counterfactual premise that causation – here etiogenesis – is a phenomenon (instead of being a noumenon). If this were the case, attention would focus on the cases preceded by the risk factor in its index category; and note would be taken of the proportion of these cases such that the antecedent actually was etiogenetic to the case. Structurally, the essence of the study would be such a restricted case series together with the documentation in it of the etiogenetic proportion for the factor at issue, proportion specific to cases occurring in association with the factor, the index category of the risk factor.

The challenge that arises from etiogenesis actually being but a noumenon is the need to provide for the case series being a manifestation (phenomenal) of the etiogenesis at issue, in terms of the etiogenetic proportion of interest (cf. above). This means that the case series is to serve documentation of rates of the outcome's occurrence in a defined study base – index and reference rates in it – conditionally on extraneous determinants of the outcome's rate of occurrence. This implies the *essence (structural) of an etiogenetic study*, including the measure of the etiogenetic proportion that it involves (as an implication of the rate ratio).

This essence of the study, in turn, implies the generic *process* to produce it, starting from the commitment to a particular source population, whether defined directly or as the catchment population of the way in which the initial (pre-reduction) case series is derived. A bit more specifically, the initial commitment is to a source population-time, to a source base, that is; and the final phase of the process now generally is the fitting of a logistic probability function to the data (now in the form of realizations for statistical variates).

While this essence, structural and procedural, of an etiogenetic study is dictated by logic, it is necessary for the students to also learn about two related concepts: that of '*cohort study*,' as this was adopted as a matter of misguided use of intervention-prognostic experiments as paradigmatic for non-experimental etiogenetic studies [9]; and that of '*case-control study*,' as this misguidedly was adopted as the solution to the feasibility problems in 'cohort studies' on rare illnesses [9]. Critical in this is the exposition of the respective fallacies, and how the correction of these leads to the singular essence of etiogenetic studies.

The common involvement of *logistic regression* in the etiogenetic study and also in the 'case-control study,' and the common use of *Cox regression* in the 'cohort study,' calls for addressing the concepts of – and in – these two types of regression, at this point in this course.

Now the students are ready to learn, concretely, *the duality in causality-oriented, directly practice-serving studies* in medicine, that constituted by the etiogenetic/etiognostic study on one side and the intervention-prognostic study on the other side [9]. The students learn that not only is the logic-dictated etiogenetic/etiognostic study not patterned after the intervention-prognostic study; it serves as a paradigm for an important aspect of RCTs, to transform the RCT from a study addressing a 'hazard ratio' (single-valued) to one producing a prognostic (intervention-prognostic) probability function (empirical) – with the involvement of logistic, rather than Cox, regression.

Once the students have a secure understanding of the essence of *the* etiogenetic study, they are ready – and they need – to learn about the principal use of this study – about *testing of etiogenetic hypotheses*. They need to learn the difference between the statistical and scientific conceptions of hypothesis and, especially, the difference between frequentist-statistical hypothesis-testing and the scientific matter of testing etiogenetic hypotheses. Important in this is, among other things, getting to understand that scientific testing ends with the evidence (original or derivative) it produces, leaving inference – the final stage in the production of scientific knowledge – to the relevant scientific community to engage in.

This use of the evidence from an etiogenetic study leads to consideration of the quality of it, the degree to which the result of the study is free from *bias*. The concepts of the three fundamental types of potential bias in an etiogenetic study need to be introduced. Given that this triad is not generally well-understood, learning it should not be impeded by the distraction of cataloguing subtypes of these.

Meant by 'the result' that may be biased in an etiogenetic hypothesis-testing study is, principally at least, the *empirical value* – single – it produces, or produced, for the rate ratio pertaining to the causal contrast at issue. This value – a 'statistic' – is the product, ultimately, of a statistical procedure, involving logistic regression, stratification, or both (in stratification by a confounder score). These procedures need to be introduced. And it is important to underscore that the rate-ratio's thus-obtained empirical value is not a 'point estimate' of the RR.

Coupled with the result of an etiogenetic hypothesis-testing study commonly is a measure of its imprecision. The students need to learn what replication-distributional properties an interval measure of this is supposed to have, the principal ways in which it is obtained, and – very importantly – that 'interval estimate' and 'confidence interval' are misnomers for this measure.

Also commonly coupled with the result of these studies is a *null P-value*. As with an interval measure of imprecision, the students need to learn what distributional properties the null P-value is supposed to have, and what are the principal ways of deriving this statistic from the data. The teacher may very well criticize the term and concept of 'testing statistical significance,' but (s)he must not make the error of questioning the role of hypothesis-testing in statistical science.

From testing etiogenetic hypotheses the teaching naturally moves to studies for *quantification* of an etiogenetic effect. For orientation to this, the students already are quite well prepared to receive the point that these studies do not produce estimates (point or interval) but only evidence for estimation (inferential, by members of the relevant scientific community).

As estimation, different from hypothesis-testing, is quantification, it presupposes *specificity* about that which is the object of the quantification. At issue here is specificity in respect to the contrasted etiogenetic histories, for one. But in addition, distinctions need to be made among subdomains of the overall domain of the study, based on potential modifiers of the RR's magnitude. This leads the teacher to address the expressions of these specificities in the log-linear model for the incidence density of the illness, in the domain of the study, the model that implies for $\log(RR)$ as a function of those particulars. At issue in this is specifics of the study's object design, bearing on its methods design (of the particulars within the study's a-priori essence, structural and procedural).

For the students to be able to rise above all of these particulars (even if only introductory) of research on the etiogenesis of illness, it is good, I think, of the teacher to delineate (the broadest particulars of) what characterizes a good etiognostic study – as to its implications for the advancement of the knowledge-base of community-level preventive medicine. For, this has bearing on the students' decisions about whether this line of research indeed will be what their future careers will be about.

As one notable alternative to epidemiological – generally etiogenetic – research in the students' career plans is meta-epidemiological clinical research, it is good, I think, of the teacher to introduce the students to the essence of research for *clinical diagnosis* – genuine essence, with a central role, again, for logistic regression. This, it needs to become clear, is in sharp contrast to what now is being taught, and practiced, by 'clinical epidemiologists' [16].

The other alternative to consider is *garnering the existing tacit knowledge* of diagnostic and prognostic experts of clinical medicine in the form of probability functions for codification in expert systems, to guide clinical practices in the interest of both quality-assurance and cost-containment in the framework of quasi-scientific medicine.

In closing, I note that a student with a solid, maximally logical orientation to epidemiological and meta-epidemiological clinical research may not have a more successful career than the one who is taught to appreciate 'cohort studies' and 'case-control studies,' and diagnostic tests' 'sensitivity' and 'specificity,' etc. (S)he may not end up with more publications, but (s)he most assuredly will make more *contributions* to the advancement of the knowledge-base of medicine. (Yes, there is 'epidemiological' research with purposes other than those noted above, but they do not belong in an introductory course on 'epidemiological' research.)